Rhetoric of the Opioid Epidemic

Lexington Studies in Contemporary Rhetoric

Series Editor: Gary C. Woodward, The College of New Jersey

This series provides thought-provoking and accessible analyses of the uses of language and media from the middle of the twentieth century to the present. In particular, this series examines how modern discourse is constructed and communicated in our distracted times, focusing on specific settings such as health communication, crisis communication, changing norms of interpersonal exchange, political communication beyond the presidency, etiquettes of communication in the digital age, celebrity as a rhetorical form, changing norms in "reality" and narrative television, and altered patterns of address in computer-mediated discussion. These books will provide depth and clarity about discourse more familiar than understood.

Recent Titles in This Series

Rhetoric of the Opioid Epidemic: Deaths of Despair in America by Tiara K. Good

A Rhetoric of Ruins: Exploring Landscapes of Abandoned Modernity by Andrew F. Wood

The Corruption of Ethos in Fortress America: Billionaires, Bodycams, and Bureaucrats by Christopher Carter

Rhetoric and Governance under Trump: Proclamations from the Bullshit Pulpit by Bernd Kaussler, Lars J. Kristiansen, and Jeffrey Delbert

Rhetorics Haunting the National Mall: Displaced and Ephemeral Public Memories edited by Roger C. Aden

Rethinking Communication in Social Business: How Re-Modeling Communication Keeps Companies Social and Entrepreneurial by Craig E. Mattson

World War I, Mass Death, and the Birth of the Modern US Soldier: A Rhetorical History by David W. Seitz

US Public Memory, Rhetoric, and the National Mall edited by Roger C. Aden

Rhetoric of the Opioid Epidemic

Deaths of Despair in America

Tiara K. Good

LEXINGTON BOOKS
Lanham • Boulder • New York • London

Published by Lexington Books
An imprint of The Rowman & Littlefield Publishing Group, Inc.
4501 Forbes Boulevard, Suite 200, Lanham, Maryland 20706
www.rowman.com

86-90 Paul Street, London EC2A 4NE

British Library Cataloguing in Publication Information Available

Library of Congress Cataloging-in-Publication Data

Names: Good, Tiara K., 1985- author.
Title: Rhetoric of the opioid epidemic : deaths of despair in America / Tiara K. Good.
Description: Lanham : Lexington Books, [2022] | Series: Lexington studies in contemporary rhetoric | Includes bibliographical references and index.
Identifiers: LCCN 2021039022 (print) | LCCN 2021039023 (ebook) | ISBN 9781793626196 (cloth) | ISBN 9781793626202 (epub)
Subjects: LCSH: Opioid abuse--United States. | Drug abuse--United States.
Classification: LCC RC568.O45 G66 2022 (print) | LCC RC568.O45 (ebook) | DDC 362.29/30973--dc23
LC record available at https://lccn.loc.gov/2021039022
LC ebook record available at https://lccn.loc.gov/2021039023

To Magnus, my lionheart who makes the world wonderful.

Contents

Acknowledgments ix

Introduction: Rhetoric of the Opioid Epidemic 1

Chapter 1: What is the Opioid Epidemic?: A Brief Summary 17

Chapter 2: Tattered Social Fabric and Dashed Expectations: Documenting the Epidemic through Documentary Films 25

Chapter 3: *Ben is Back*: Mothers of the Epidemic 47

Chapter 4: Defining Trump's America through Crisis: Remarks on Combating the Opioid Crisis 63

Chapter 5: Mapping the Epidemic: ODMAP and the Boundaries of Response 87

Chapter 6: A Brief Analysis and Sample of the Chronic Pain Management Debate in the United States 107

Conclusion: A Very American Epidemic: Rhetoric of the Opioid Epidemic 121

Bibliography 131

Index 137

About the Author 139

Acknowledgments

Thank you to Nicolette, my editor, for your patience and walking me through my first book writing experience. A hearty nod to the rigorous training at The Pennsylvania State University Communication Arts and Sciences department to prepare me for such an endeavor. Dr. Jeremy Engels and Dr. Brad Vivian stand out as two who were supportive and continue to reach out from time to time to keep me on my scholarly toes.

Thank you to my Magnus for being with me throughout the whole process. Such a patient little one while I wrote, edited, and rambled on about things to you. One day you will be old enough to read this and watch the films with me.

Random chats about the topic, a bit of levity when I needed a break from the topic, letting me bounce ideas around, and your eyes to edit—grateful for my friends who supplied the aforementioned.

Introduction

Rhetoric of the Opioid Epidemic

Since the late 1990s, the opioid epidemic has been a uniquely American phenomenon. Fueled by prescription pain medications, the opioid epidemic has been one of the most devastating public health crises the United States has ever seen. About twenty years prior, Purdue Pharma created a unique metric by introducing pain as a "quality of life" measure. As a result, doctors started screening their patients using this measure which led to the idea that pain should be eliminated altogether.[1] Dr. Sanjay Gupta reports that "As of 2011, 75% of the world's opioid prescription drugs are prescribed and swallowed up in a country that makes up less than 5% of the world's population, leading to the most common cause of unintentional death in America today—drug overdose."[2] The Centers for Disease Control and Prevention (CDC) points to the beginning of the epidemic starting in 1999 and describes it as developing in three waves: from 1999 with the increase of prescription opioids to treat pain, from 2010 with "rapid increases in overdose deaths involving heroin," and from 2013 with "significant increases in overdose deaths involving synthetic opioids."[3]

By the second wave, the opioid epidemic had become more visible in popular culture, and was picking up speed with governmental responses and politics. Popular television series, *Nurse Jackie,* won Edie Falco an Emmy for Best Actress and the series for "Outstanding Comedy Series" in 2010.[4] It was a popular television series that highlighted the struggles of an individual with opioid use disorder (OUD), to its credit, in 2009 when the topic was largely ignored. But it was billed as a comedy and missed the mark as far as digging into the epidemic. After 2009, there was a lag before more television series and films started taking up the opioid epidemic writ large or even the topic of an individual. The next large and visible moment publicly in the epidemic timeline comes in 2016, with President Obama proclaiming, "During Prescription Opioid and Heroin Epidemic Awareness Week, we pause to remember all those we have lost to OUD, we stand with the courageous individuals in recovery, and we recognize the importance of raising awareness of this epidemic."[5] The Obama administration added funding for: evidence-based prevention programs, prescription drug monitoring, prescription drug take-back events, medication-assisted treatment, and the overdose reversal drug naloxone.

Records show that 2017 was one of the deadliest years in the opioid epidemic. That was the same year that the Department of Health and Human Services (HHS) declared the epidemic a public health emergency.[6] The Trump administration claimed the prior administration did not do enough on this issue and declared the opioid epidemic a "public health emergency" in October 2017.[7] This book focuses on the years surrounding 2017—the deadliest year in the epidemic—and offers case studies that demonstrate the governmental and mediated responses to the opioid epidemic.

In this book, I engage texts through a rhetorical lens to better understand discursive formations and patterns about the opioid epidemic. My goal is to start to understand the vocabulary of the epidemic. How we talk about things matters. How they are represented is important. In order to achieve this goal, I analyze case studies from popular culture and governmental responses to the opioid epidemic. The case studies include two documentaries,*Heroin(e)* (2017) and *One Nation Under Stress: Deaths of Despair in the United States* (2019); *Ben is Back* (2018); President Trump's March 19, 2018, address to the nation; the Drug Enforcement Agency's High-Intensity Drug Trafficking Areas (HIDTA) ODMAP; and news stories from national sources dating from 2015 to 2020 about the chronic pain management debate. I adjust my methodology and approach throughout the book to fit the text being analyzed in particular chapters, but will have the overarching Burkean synecdoche underlying my analysis throughout the book. Burke defines a synecdoche as a "representation" and a "part for the whole."[8] By understanding representative parts of the rhetoric and discourses of the opioid epidemic, we may glean better insights about the broader whole. Brief literature reviews and relevant context to the texts are given in every analytical chapter. My wish is not to be exhaustive in my analysis, but to provide an initial foray into this complex and dynamic landscape of the opioid epidemic for students and scholars alike. Ultimately, it would be excellent were it to pique the curiosity and research venture of my fellow communication scholars. The greatest outcome of this book would be to encourage other books to be written that further analyze the opioid epidemic and other areas of deaths of despair. There is an enormous scope and scale involved that one book cannot possibly cover.

OPIOIDS: A VERY DIFFERENT EPIDEMIC

The outrageous rates of opioid use and sheer death toll—significant enough to cause a trend of decreased life expectancy in a particular demographic—make the opioid epidemic stand apart from prior epidemics. It stands apart in a few key ways: actions taken by the government, the public's response to a matter involving drug use in the United States, and rhetorical responses. The latter two have been strikingly different. It seems as though the shift to a public health frame and medicalization narratives, with an emphasis on it being an epidemic, came early and while the epidemic is still an ongoing crisis. Most often, by public health experts and doctors, the opioid epidemic is compared to the AIDS epidemic of the 1980s because that had been the deadliest epidemic before the opioid epidemic. "Not since the HIV/AIDS epidemic has the United States faced as devastating and lethal a health problem as the current crisis of opioid misuse and overdose and OUD. Current national trends indicate that each year more people die of overdoses—the majority of which involve opioid drugs—than died in the entirety of the Vietnam War, the Korean War, or any armed conflict since the end of World War II."[9] Case and Deaton use two epidemics—the crack cocaine and HIV/AIDS epidemics—which precede the opioid epidemic and occurred simultaneously in the 1980s as comparative epidemics.[10] Both had high death rates. Troubling and apathetic governmental responses as well as the public's poor opinion of the victims involved in these two epidemics make them apt reference points of comparison. With each of the prior epidemics, the public viewed individuals involved as those with a bad moral compass or as outright deviant and derelict people who deserved to be punished for their shortcomings and choices. Next, I offer some background on how the rhetorical and public responses were for the AIDS epidemic and some case studies that communication scholars have noted.

The HIV/AIDS epidemic was first viewed, not as a public health issue or an epidemic, but as punishment for particular communities deemed undesirable. Marita Sturken writes, "the person contaminated with AIDS was from the beginning considered a figure of sexual deviancy and threat. Even more than the leper or the syphilitic, the person with AIDS was perceived to be socially irresponsible and hedonistic, who sacrificed life and health for perverse pleasure with strangers."[11] The 1980s were rife with crime-centric policies and an aversion to otherized communities, such as the gay community, and initial public policies for dealing with containment of the disease included registries and exclusion of children suffering from the disease from schools. In spite of high numbers of infection rates in IV-drug and hemophilia sufferers, AIDS was most identified with gay men in the 1980s and early 1990s in the media and politically as the opposite of "family values" and detrimental to the security of life in America. Sturken remarks, "AIDS emerged early and devastatingly in urban gay communities, which predominantly comprise middle-class professionals. From the beginning, AIDS was associated in this country with practices regarded as deviant (homosexuality, drug use, sexual promiscuity)."[12] That same group most visibly identified with AIDS was also one of the groups that had a "sophisticated understanding of media and marketing" and was able to begin the hard work of shifting representations of AIDS to a public health epidemic, rather than a curse of deviance and support for right-wing, punitive policies.[13]

While I do not delve into the sociological and economic underlying causes elsewhere in the book, I find that it is important to note the inequity, quick attention, and kinder rhetorical framing that the opioid epidemic receives compared to epidemics in the past. Because the epidemic was first noted in a white population, that certainly plays a role in the attention, types of attention, funding, rhetorical framing, and concern the opioid epidemic has garnered. The rhetorical work of using an epidemic metaphor early in the understanding and development of opioid use in the United States, I argue, helped shape approaches to the epidemic. Using this health framing early in understanding, and defining what was occurring, drives much of how opioid use is met by the public, media, and policy makers.

I refer to the use of epidemic as a metaphor due to the complexity of the issue. Epidemics are typically associated with a rapidly infectious disease. The opioid epidemic is "infectious" in a sense, due to the numerous and systemic underlying roots of the matter, but because it is not literally an infectious disease, there may be slippages in the public health frame and medicalization of the issue that are important to identify in the case studies. Lakoff and Johnson, in their book *Philosophy in the Flesh*, discuss the importance of metaphors, how they are able to take on truth value, and their transparency to human cognition. According to George Lakoff and Mark Johnson, "metaphors supply the logic, the imagery, and the qualitative feel of sensorimotor experience to abstract concepts. We all acquire these metaphorical modes of thought automatically and unconsciously and have no choice as to whether or not to use them."[14] Metaphors assist with comprehending new, abstract, and complicated concepts. Addiction as a disease and as an infectious one, as connoted in the use of the term *epidemic,* is a metaphor to an extent. This is not to refute the literal disease components that go along with addiction. There are plenty of neurobiological underpinnings to support that addiction is a disease and numerous medical studies confirm it as well. This understanding and research are not yet universally accepted in American culture and society. Even if it were, it is still a rhetorical choice—and a powerful one—to name the matter an *epidemic*. Throughout this book, I explore case studies in which the medicalization of the opioid epidemic is implemented. Part of my pursuit in analyzing these case studies is to start to develop an understanding of the motives of that work, if there are commonalities amongst the medicalization rhetoric, and identify how it is rhetorically implemented.

Proposed solutions are numerous, but stigma and misperceptions lay in the way of many of the solutions that have been put forward and ability to gain meaningful traction. The public health lens and referring to the phenomenon as an "epidemic" does important rhetorical work. Erin Willis and Chad Painter's research looking at how stories framing the opioid and heroin epidemics in the state use a health communication frame in major news outlets across Cincinnati, Ohio, sheds important light:

> Instead of applying the "war on drugs'" policies of previous decades (Duke & Gross, 2014), politicians and policymakers, at the local and national level, are treating opioid and heroin addiction as a public health problem rather than an issue of criminal justice. In recent years, policymakers have sought solutions that help reduce use and overdose by expanding access to treatment, modifying penalties, and increasing access to naloxone (National Conference of State Legislatures, 2017).[15]

There is a marked shift in much of the framing of the opioid epidemic that is moving away from the "war on drugs" approach that was so common in American rhetoric and politics. Furthermore, Willis and Painter argue, "Portrayals of public health problems and health inequalities influence the public's perception of the problem and what should be done to solve it."[16] The medicalization of the opioid epidemic eases the stigmatization that sufferers face. For years, Americans had a cultural and societal understanding that drug use was a moral failing and ultimately a choice that called for legal punishment. Michael Botticelli and Colleen L. Barry, distinguished public health policy experts, give an historical view on the issue:

> For decades, the public at large has viewed, and continues to view, addiction as simply a matter of individual choice. This view is largely driven by a lack of scientific understanding of the genetic, environmental, and neurobiologic aspects of SUDs and addiction. Those who cannot seem to "control" their behavior (which can often be distressing and highly upsetting to others) continue to be seen as weak-willed or morally flawed.[17]

Stigma is a huge hurdle for many who would seek treatment or notice they are beginning to become dependent on their prescription pain killers. Most of society has a long way to go regarding better approaches to how we even discuss and represent addiction. Botticelli and Barry argue, "Language is perpetuated by the general public, by the media, by the medical community, and even by those in the recovery community. Historically, we have used language to isolate those affected and to treat them in a less than compassionate and therapeutic way."[18] While I focus on the medicalization of the opioid epidemic, I do not assume that this representation is necessarily standardized across all instances of representation and rhetorical choices regarding opioid use. Resistance and misunderstandings about interventions in the opioid epidemic, even to access to overdose reversing medication, in some of the case studies reveal that this is not the gold-standard approach to representation nor how we colloquially communicate about opioid use.

The vocabulary of medicalization shifts the ways in which society understands those impacted by the ravages of the opioid epidemic. Medicalization is defined as "a process in which the expertise of science and medicine (and the public vocabularies that support such expertise) is valued over lived and experiential knowledge and used to categorize aspects of social life as disease or abnormality."[19] While putting the opioid crisis in terms that are medical (i.e., an epidemic), it shifts away from the older era of seeing drug crises as moral failings. Framing it as in need of a public health response has been argued to be beneficial and reduce stigma as well. It is not without a power dynamic though. There is still a potential for people suffering from OUD to be deindividualized and subject to other forms of discipline. Deborah Lupton explains, "From a Foucauldian perspective, power as it operates in the medical encounter is a disciplinary power that provides guidelines about how patients should understand, regulate and experience their bodies."[20] Discipline, in a Foucauldian sense, shifts from the institutions of law enforcement to that of healthcare and behavioral health providers.

By exploring case studies, I will demonstrate how the public health frame and naming it an epidemic, rather than a drug or crime issue, works in specific ways to reduce stigma and can assist in reshaping public perspectives. The case studies are drawn from governmental responses to the epidemic, news media reporting, and popular media representations. The discourse of an epidemic can also alleviate pressure from the individual and place it upon the collective. The epidemic frames the crisis a medical issue, not the moral failing and shortcomings of a few bad apples run amok, and holds more potential for solving the epidemic through medical treatment and reconnecting sufferers back to society. This is a rhetorical move that separates the opioid epidemic from the criminal and immoral frames that were cast upon the crack epidemic and the initial framing of the AIDS epidemic. The public health framing and medicalization narratives rhetorically demands the question: what will *we* do as a country about the epidemic?

No state, county, or city is immune to this epidemic. It is not a strictly rural or urban problem. The opioid epidemic is insidious and the underlying causes are so complex and numerous that it is hard to picture a way out of it. Kristoff and WuDunn describe the complexity and failings revealed by the opioid epidemic as a long suffering that could have been avoided:

> Suffering in working-class America was not inevitable but rather reflects decades of social-policy mistakes and often gratuitous cruelty: the war on drugs that led to mass incarceration, indifference to the loss of blue-collar jobs, insufficient health-care coverage, embrace of a highly unequal education system, tax giveaways to tycoons, zillionaire-friendly court decisions, acceptance of growing inequality, and systematic underinvestment in children and community services such as drug treatment.[21]

This problem is not a *drug* problem and the discourses surrounding the opioid epidemic are fascinating ones. By 2020, the nuance surrounding the issue is laudable in some areas and the lack of nuance is noteworthy in others. What becomes most clear is that the opioid epidemic is complicated, messy, and we are nowhere near a cogent solution as a society.

Underlying causes of the opioid epidemic come up frequently throughout the texts I will analyze. One theory in particular will surface a few times. Achenbach and Keating continue their story describing the *dashed expectations theory,* "One theory about what is causing rising mortality among whites is the 'dashed expectations' hypothesis. According to Johns Hopkins University sociologist Andrew Cherlin, whites today are more pessimistic than their forebears about their opportunities to advance in life."[22] With fewer opportunities without a four-year degree, less social support, and lower quality of life than the generations before them, Cherlin and others assert that many Americans, particularly white ones, find their lives in despair because they have not achieved what they thought they would. This is certainly not the last time the *dashed expectations theory* will appear in this book. If not explicitly by name, the theory will be explored using other terms and through numerous individual accounts of the opioid epidemic. The notion of *dashed expectations* and the unraveling of society in the United States in general are consistently part of the discourse of the opioid epidemic. The underlying causes are plentiful and not easily remedied. Because, as I mentioned already, it becomes clear that the opioid epidemic is not a drug epidemic, it is so much more than that. The opioid epidemic peeled back layers of inequity, social issues, political problems, and much more to expose underlying issues that impact the daily lives of many Americans.

Before the COVID-19 pandemic of 2020, the opioid epidemic was a major public health issue and there was no end in sight. Harmeet Kaur of CNN wrote in May 2020, shortly after the beginning of the epidemic, "Opioids account for a majority of drug overdose deaths, the leading cause of accidental death in the US. It's a crisis that's been a priority for officials at the federal, state and local levels for years.[23]" Governmental responses were varied at these different levels, but the epidemic was definitely a priority. With the pandemic, the opioid epidemic continued and even accelerated. Many individuals afflicted by COVID-19 experienced obstacles to treatment and factors that likely lead to opioid use disorders. Opioid overdoses are spiking all over the country as a result of the complicating factors of the pandemic.[24] Increased stress and anxiety, sudden joblessness, lack of support from treatment centers closing, and more have thrown the opioid epidemic a curve that has left the nation unable to balance treating both public health issues simultaneously.

A BRIEF OVERVIEW OF LITERATURE ON RHETORIC OF EPIDEMICS

While there are no full-length books from the discipline of rhetoric about the opioid epidemic, there are only a few journal articles that approach the subject. Using the search terms "rhetoric" and "opioid" only yields two journal articles in the database *Communication and Mass Media Complete.*[25] Since there are so few articles about this particular topic, I have also included literature from rhetoricians writing about the rhetoric of epidemics more broadly and health communication as it relates to the issue.

The opioid epidemic has impacted particular areas of the country with more intensity than others. There are several factors as to why certain regions see worse rates of opioid use and deaths. Part of that is the ways in which the drugs are prescribed, but furthermore, where drugs like fentanyl and heroin are more accessible and trafficked into the country. Finkelman and McGinnis point out, "While the crisis does not discriminate in terms of who or where it touches, opioid overdose deaths are most common among non-Hispanic whites, among individuals aged 25 to 54 years old, and in the Northeast, Midwest, and Southern US Census Bureau regions."[26] These are regions where drugs, like fentanyl in particular, have been more accessible. States and counties in these regions are dealing with the epidemic more acutely than others.

Not surprisingly, the journal articles that cover the opioid epidemic are focused on case studies from Philadelphia, Pennsylvania, and Ohio. Policy and approaches to the opioid epidemic are key to understanding the rhetoric of the opioid epidemic. Ashley Ferrell's article about the introduction and implementation of progressive, though highly controversial, CUES in Philadelphia highlights the inequities and gentler rhetorical choices made about the opioid epidemic versus prior epidemics. The treatment of the crack cocaine and HIV/AIDS epidemics of decades past had long-lasting and devastating effects on African American and Latinx communities in Philadelphia.

Ferrell finds, "A key component of positioning Philadelphia's present rash of overdoses as a public health issue entailed presenting opioid addiction as a disease as opposed to a deficit of individual ethics, a moral failing, and a punishable offense, as was common in the recent past treatment of those engaging in substance use."[27] She points to the "war on drugs" policies of the past, and blatant racism, which were hueing the ways in which prior epidemics were treated and talked about as highly problematic. The historical moment of in which the CUES were presented allowed for a kairotic moment "allowed the community to reveal racialized ideologies lining the discursive framing of this harm reduction intervention."[28] Media treatment and framing are also essential for understanding the rhetoric of the opioid epidemic.

Framing lends tremendous insights about how we understand, relate to, and evaluate situations. David Russell, Kelly M. Thames, and Naomi J. Spence researched the ways in which newspapers in Ohio and citizens of Ohio's posted to their Facebook pages. Russel et al. illuminate the importance of media treatment and framing as well as cultural assumptions here, "While media organizations frame how drug epidemics are presented to the public, audience views are also shaped by dominant cultural beliefs and attitudes towards drug use. Americans frequently possess stigmatizing beliefs about opioid use that favor punitive policies and lesser support for public health interventions (Kennedy-Hendricks et al., 2017)."[29] Their study found that most newspapers were reporting about the epidemic in a denigrating way that emphasized criminality and law enforcement approaches. Public health frames were not as prevalent and when present, tended to be more contextualized than the criminality frames used. Of the criminality frames present, Russel et al. note, "Some of this reporting, especially stories with minimal context or investigative resources may promote stigmatization of opioid use."[30] While my focus is on the public health framing and medicalization of the epidemic, it is important to understand that examples of criminality frames are still found. Public health framing and the medicalization of the opioid epidemic reflect the enormous amount of cultural and perceptual work has to do to work against the stigmatized and older perceptions about drug use. Willis and Painter remark, "America's view of health should be one of broad social perspective, not one that focuses on individual factors. Journalists should consider using news frames that begin to shift the cultural narrative away from focusing on individuals and their personal behaviors to the community's health and how individuals can be part of the greater solution."[31]

The rhetoric of epidemics has received more treatment from rhetoricians. Ebola, HIV/AIDS, and obesity have all been written about. Of epidemics broadly with a focus on governmental responses, Nancy Roth's article illustrates, "the rhetorical association of epidemic disease with groups perceived to be *other* performs a distancing function that allows healthy groups to see themselves as separate from those who are unhealthy."[32] Much like the dis-identification with the present opioid epidemic that Philadelphians promoted in Ferrell's piece, epidemics can have a distancing effect rhetorically. Roth finds that governmental rhetoric about epidemics emphasize, "the importance of individual behavioral change as a health strategy can be attributed to the government's need to cut costs in the face of a recession and spiraling medical costs in the nineteen seventies and eighties. Over the course of those years, the government changed its health policy from one of providing access to more comprehensive services to one of cost control."[33] Cost control and individual agency are both prominent in the discourse of epidemics.

How to shift individual actions and perceptions about approaches is another goal of the rhetoric of epidemics. Celeste Condit's article about the Ebola epidemic and most recent outbreak that reached the United States focused on the ways in which public health officials succeed and fail to get their messages across to the public. Condit posits that there was a decline in public faith in public health officials that "an exacerbation of the inherent gap between experts and publics" after the 2014–2015 Ebola outbreak. Furthermore, Condit argues, "To do their work, public health messages must be taken up by members of the public or at least their representatives, and publics have good reason not to automatically cede their judgments to experts merely because they claim expertise."[34] Public health officials and policy lacking the ethos necessary to shift a public's perceptions and gain buy-in for changing attitudes as well as behaviors is devastating in the fight of an epidemic. The HIV/AIDS epidemic around the globe receives mixed approaches from public health officials and administrations. Shaping public perceptions of those approaches are complex and fraught with tension, but one study suggests that the rhetorical choices can have great influence on acceptance of approaches and funding. Franklin Nii Amankwah Yartey found that, "Funding for HIV/AIDS increased drastically between 2002 and 2008; during this time period the disease was framed as a national security threat" (Baringer & Heitkamp 2011). Furthermore, Yartey asserts this framing is continued because, "the securitization of HIV/AIDS . . . draws attention and funding to suffering populations experiencing weak economics and deteriorating defenses due to the scourge of HIV/AIDS."[35] This affirms the argument that framing a health issue as a security threat mobilizes support and aid for that health issue."[36] The securitization framing of public health assists with justifying framing when an entire body politic views the funds as helping them personally stay safe against the threat of an epidemic.

In the findings about the rhetoric of the obesity epidemic in the United States, personal action and agency are most prevalent and has strong correlations to the opioid epidemic. Sonia R. Ivancic's study of the proposed soda ban reveals much about public health policy and the ways in which it does not mix well with American culture. Ivancic observes of the discourses surrounding the soda ban:

> These discourses surface a noteworthy tension in the conventional neoliberal imaginary which is predicated on the state collaboratively facilitating industry, always privileging the market's interests. While governments benefit from productive yet consuming citizens, industry stands to benefit enormously from obesity through the profit generated from consuming citizens (who may or may not become fat) and from the "obesity epidemic" itself.[37]

Similarly, to how corporations—such as pharmaceutical companies and even doctors to an extent—benefited enormously from the profits gained from opioid pain killers, those taking the pills were likely to get worse, addicted, and then become viewed as more costly citizens to the government.

Epidemics, such as the obesity and opioid epidemics, that have perceptions that include discourses of choice and individual agency face unique challenges. Ivancic finds that health discourses around epidemics that include consumption demonstrate, "how these 'unhealthy' bodies are a communal (national) concern, these body liability discourses position fit and 'cheap' bodies as good, patriotic citizens."[38] There is a risk with the public health frame being presented in economic terms rather than a citizen's right to health. Emma Frances Bloomfield and Angeline Sangalang's article about popular documentaries tackling the obesity epidemic yielded similar insights to Ivancic's. Bloomfield and Sangalang observe a political and cultural split in the public perception, "Conservatives are consequently more likely to find blame for acts in an individual's actions and behaviors. In the health debate, assigning responsibility to the agent often implies empowering individuals to make choices regarding their health without regulations," while Liberals hold the "scene" more accountable than the individual. Thus, "exonerating the agent from complete responsibility. In the health debate, assigning responsibility to the scene often implies government regulation on industry."[39] Depending on where the rhetorical emphasis lies, public perceptions and expectations of approaches can be influenced tremendously.

ARRANGEMENT OF THE BOOK

In this book, I delve into various popular and governmental responses to the epidemic. Each case study is a representative anecdote of the main, critical areas to the opioid epidemic. The following chapters focus on specific texts, either from a popular source or governmental agency, but engages themes that persist throughout the broader rhetorical formation of this issue as an epidemic. I have defined the main and critical areas of the opioid epidemic as popular and governmental because both are vital for understanding how the public perceives the epidemic. Representative anecdotes, according to Kenneth Burke, are a "reduction" of something in the pursuit to "seek for vocabularies that will be faithful *reflections* of reality."[40] Furthermore, a representative anecdote may be "used as a form in conformity with which the vocabulary is constructed."[41] Meaning, since I cannot exhaustively cover all aspects of representation of the opioid epidemic, the case studies I analyze will yield a representation of the overall whole of the discourses, or *vocabulary,* of the opioid epidemic. I find it essential to analyze texts that are derived from both governmental and popular culture sources. Both have profound influence and can impact the course of approaches to an epidemic.

How the epidemic is talked about, why it is referred to as an *epidemic,* and the frames used while presenting and representing the epidemic are all questions I seek to answer. Additionally, through rhetorical analysis of popular culture and governmental responses, how the opioid epidemic altered and reshaped narratives of drug abuse and overdose deaths will be a pursuit of the book. Now, with the medicalized narratives and public health framing of the opioid epidemic, drug addicts are more likely to look like a white, middle-class, grandmother. Drug dealers are now visualized as white coat wearing M.D.s with prescription pads.

Additionally, I tried to write the book in an accessible way that can be read by undergraduate classes from multiple disciplines. I do not dive into heavy rhetorical theory and spend most of my analysis pursuits pulling at the larger trends and themes. By analyzing and understanding what some of the larger themes are, we will gain a better understanding of how the epidemic is being represented. Gaining a vocabulary of the epidemic offers more insight into how we as a society understand and approach the epidemic and those affected by it. To the best of my knowledge, this book is the first of its kind to focus on the rhetoric of the opioid epidemic. There are many fantastic books and research articles about defining deaths of despair, the opioid epidemic, underlying causes, statistics, general information, and possible solutions. If you are looking for books that cover that material in-depth, this is not that book. I hope the following chapters provide further insight into the ways in which we visualize, talk about, debate about, and the government responds to the opioid epidemic.

OUTLINE OF CHAPTERS

To study the rhetoric of this issue is to ultimately argue that the discourses surrounding it did not have to shape it into something called an epidemic. Like the "war on drugs," this issue could have gone the same road and shared a similar rhetorical fate as prolific and devastating use of crack cocaine in the 1980s. In order to see why and how opioids are treated differently, I tend to texts from official governmental agencies, news media, and popular realms. Each area influences the perceptions of American society and culture in important ways and are critical to gaining insights into the discursive shape of how this epidemic is represented as such. The rhetorical ways in which discourses are formed are crucial for understanding how we as a society understand something and how we arrived at that understanding. The first chapter is a brief summary of the opioid epidemic to provide context and background for the analysis chapters. This is not an exhaustive chapter about every aspect of the opioid epidemic, but a brief read to prepare for the analyses to follow.

The book is divided into two parts. I begin by looking at popular media representations of the opioid epidemic. I then turn my focus to governmental responses to the opioid epidemic. The first section of the book analyzes popular media texts. Chapter 2 is titled "Tattered Social Fabric and Dashed Expectations: Documenting the Epidemic through Documentary Films." This chapter is a rhetorical analysis of two documentaries: *Heroin(e)* and *One Nation Under Stress: Deaths of Despair in the United States.* Both are award-winning documentaries and examine different facets of the opioid epidemic. I find the two offer a well-rounded perspective on deaths of despair, the opioid epidemic in particular, and are plentiful for rhetorical analysis. Chapter 3, titled "*Ben is Back*: Mothers of the Epidemic," is a close-textual analysis of a major motion film directed by Peter Hedges. It is one of the only Hollywood films about the opioid epidemic and features a star-filled cast and award-winning director. Themes and framing of the epidemic within the film are also explored in this chapter. *Ben is Back* is one of the few major motion picture films that focuses exclusively on the opioid epidemic.

In the second section, I sought out case studies that would be impactful to legislation and the technology involved in responding to the epidemic. Since governmental communication and responses to the epidemic are plentiful, I chose case studies that would reflect high-level decision-making as well as interesting cases of technology developed by government agencies in order to approach the epidemic. Chapter 4, titled "Defining Trump's America through Crisis: Remarks on Combatting the Opioid Crisis," is a close-textual analysis of President Trump's March 19, 2018, address to the nation. I explore themes and frames deployed throughout the speech to define the epidemic as well as the President's vision of the nation. Chapter 5, titled "Mapping the Epidemic: ODMAP and the Boundaries of Response," is rhetorical analysis of the visual and textual facets of the ODMAP produced by the Washington/Baltimore High Intensity Drug Trafficking Area unit. The technology is used by law enforcement, first responders, public health officials, and governmental organizations all over the United States. Chapter 6, titled "A Brief Analysis and Sample of the Chronic Pain Management Debate in the United States," is a media framing analysis of news stories from 2015 to 2020 about the chronic pain management debate as it pertains to the opioid epidemic.

Due to the multifaceted and complex nature of the opioid epidemic, I selected case studies to analyze that would cover various areas of response to the epidemic. Areas included are: policy and legislation, technology, sources that inform, national debate, and popular media sources that move audiences. Each area is a representative anecdote, a part of the whole, of a complicated and multilayered epidemic. Overall, my analysis seeks answers to the following questions and inform about the vocabulary of the opioid epidemic: Why and how does this particular moment in time enable the medicalization and public health framing of this issue? Is it consistent? If not, where and how do those slippages in the rhetoric occur? I argue that the rhetoric of the opioid epidemic has been vastly medicalized and framed through public health in order to garner support for policies and approaches that will be more effective than the epidemics of the past in most cases. By presenting it as a health issue—not as individuals with moral failings, drug problems, and poor decision-making skills—it puts the responsibility of approaches to the issue upon the collective and demands the government to regulate the systems that lead to the epidemic proportions of the problem. It also demands a cultural and broader economic shift that does not reward corporate greed with the lives of our citizens. Furthermore, the rhetoric of the "war on drugs" has not been shrug entirely and the work of these novel rhetorical choices of naming the issue an *epidemic* early, medicalization, and the public health frame still have more perceptual and cultural work ahead. I will demonstrate how the rhetorical ghosts of the "war on drugs" and criminal framing of prior drug issues in America are still haunting the immense amount of progress yet to be made in the stymying of this epidemic and change of perception helpful to its healthful conclusion.

NOTES

1. Anna Lembke, M.D., *Drug Dealer, MD: How Doctors Were Duped, Patients Got Hooked, and Why It's So Hard to Stop* (Baltimore: Johns Hopkins University Press, 2016), 3.

2. Dr. Sanjay Gupta, "Doctors Must Lead Us out of Our Opioid Abuse Epidemic," *CNN,* June 2, 2016, https://www.cnn.com/2016/05/11/health/sanjay-gupta-prescription-addiction-doctors-must-lead/index.html.

3. "Understanding the Epidemic," *Centers for Disease Control,* March 19, 2020, https://www.cdc.gov/drugoverdose/epidemic/index.html.

4. "Nurse Jackie," *Emmy's,* https://www.emmys.com/shows/nurse-jackie.

5. President Barack Obama, "Fact Sheet: Obama Administration Announces Prescription Opioid and Heroin Epidemic Awareness Week," September 19, 2016, https://obamawhitehouse.archives.gov/the-press-office/2016/09/19/fact-sheet-obama-administration-announces-prescription-opioid-and-heroin.

6. "What is the U.S. Opioid Epidemic?," *Department of Health and Human Services,* February 19, 2021, https://www.hhs.gov/opioids/about-the-epidemic/index.html.

7. "Ending America's Opioid Crisis," Whitehouse.gov, 2020, https://www.whitehouse.gov/opioids/.

8. Ibid, 507–508.

9. Richard J. Bonnie, "Trends in Opioid Use, Harms, and Treatment." In *Pain Management and the Opioid Epidemic: Balancing Societal and Individual Benefits and Risks of Prescription Opioid Use* (Washington D.C.: The National Academies Press) 188.

10. Anne Case and Angus Deaton, *Deaths of Despair and the Future of Capitalism* (New Jersey: Princeton University Press, 2020), 5.

11. Marita Sturken, *Tangled Memories: The Vietnam War, the AIDS Epidemic, and the Politics of Remembering* (Berkeley: University of California Press, 1997) 150.

12. Ibid, 145.

13. Ibid, 146.

14. George Lakoff and Mark Johnson, *Philosophy in the Flesh* (New York, New York: Basic Books, 1999) 128.

15. Erin Willis and Chad Painter, "The Needle and the Damage Done: Framing the Heroin Epidemic in the Cincinnati Enquirer," *Health Communication* 34 (6), (2019): 661.

16. Ibid, 662.

17. Michael Botticelli and Colleen L. Barry, "Stigma and the Language of Addiction." In *A Public Health Guide to Ending the Opioid Epidemic*, edited by Jay C. Butler, and Michael R. Fraser (Oxford University Press, 2019) 34.

18. Ibid, 39.

19. Robin E. Jensen, "Improving Upon Nature: The Rhetorical Ecology of Chemical Language, Reproductive Endocrinology, and the Medicalization of Infertility," *Quarterly Journal of Speech* 101 (2), (2015): 330.

20. Deborah Lupton, "Foucault and the Medicalisation Critique." In *Foucault, Health and Medicine*, edited by Alan Petersen and Robin Bunton (London: Routledge, 1997) 99.

21. Nicholas D. Kristof and Sheryl WuDunn, *Tightrope: Americans Reaching for Hope* (New York: Alfred A. Knopf, 2020) 18.

22. Ibid.

23. Harmeet Kaur, "The Opioid Epidemic was Already a National Crisis. COVID-19 Could be Making Things Worse," *CNN*, May 7, 2020, https://www.cnn.com/2020/05/07/health/opioid-epidemic-covid19-pandemic-trnd/index.html.

24. Ibid.

25. Communication and Mass Media Complete is the "go to" database for the rhetoric discipline.

26. Elizabeth M. Finkelman and J. Michael McGinnis, "The Emergence of an Epidemic." In *A Public Health Guide to Ending the Opioid Epidemic*, edited by Jay C. Butler and Michael R. Fraser (Oxford: Oxford University Press, 2019), 7.

27. Ashley P. Ferrell, "'Righting Past Wrongs': Rhetorical Disidentification and Historical Reference in Response to Philadelphia's Opioid Epidemic," *Rhetoric & Public Affairs* 22 (4), (2019): 550–51.

28. Ibid, 556.

29. David Russell, Kelly M. Thames, and Naomi J. Spence, "'It's So Scary How Common This Is Now': Frames in Media Coverage of the Opioid Epidemic by Ohio Newspapers and Themes in Facebook User Reactions." *Information, Communication & Society* 22 (5), (2019): 703.

30. Ibid, 707.

31. Erin Willis and Chad Painter, "The Needle and the Damage Done: Framing the Heroin Epidemic in the Cincinnati Enquirer," *Health Communication* 34 (6), (2019): 667.

32. Nancy L. Roth, "Dismantling the Mosaic of Misery: Louis Sullivan's Paradoxic Rhetorical Vision," *Howard Journal of Communications* 4 (3), (1993): 235.

33. Ibid, 245.

34. Celeste M. Condit, "Public Health Experts, Expertise, and Ebola: A Relational Theory of Ethos," *Rhetoric & Public Affairs* 22 (2), (2019): 204–205.

35. Franklin Nii Amankwah Yartey, "The Critical Condition of Rhetorical Choices," *Journal of International Communication* 21 (2), (2015): 2229.

36. Ibid, 234.

37. Sonia R. Ivancic, "Body Sovereignty and Body Liability in the Wake of an 'Obesity Epidemic': A Poststructural Analysis of the Soda Ban," *Health Communication* 33 (10), (2018): 1253.

38. Ibid, 1250.

39. Emma Frances Bloomfield and Angeline Sangalang, "Juxtaposition as Visual Argument: Health Rhetoric in Super Size Me and Fat Head," *Argumentation & Advocacy* 50 (3), (2014): 144.

40. Kenneth Burke, *A Grammar of Motives* (Berkeley: The University of California Press, 1969) 59.

41. Ibid, 59.

Chapter 1

What is the Opioid Epidemic?

A Brief Summary

The opioid epidemic death rate is alarming. According to the *Centers for Disease Control*, "128 people die every day from an opioid overdose."[1] The impact is so severe, it is causing age expectancy rates in the United States to decline for the first time since World War I.[2] Deaths of Despair is a term coined by Anne Case. These deaths are defined by opioid overdose, suicide, and alcohol-related deaths, and they are now the leading causes of death in the United States. Anne Case and Angus Deaton, economists out of Princeton University, explain the term here, "deaths of despair come from a long-standing process of cumulative disadvantage for those with less than a college degree."[3] Their research revealed a startling trend of life expectancy decreasing in the United States for the first time since the early 1900s. Case and Deaton's observation that non-Hispanic whites in America were dying at disproportional rates of deaths of despair, with opioid overdoses being the bulk of the cause of death, was revelatory. The lynchpin in their study shows that the most predominant factor of opioid deaths was education level. "The widening gap between those with and without a bachelor's degree is not only in death but also in quality of life; those without a degree are seeing increases in their levels of pain, ill health, and serious mental distress, and declines in their ability to work and socialize," remark Case and Deaton.[4] They have found that deaths of despair impact those with "less than a college degree" most notably. Education being a key factor to this equation starts to reveal a significant shortcoming to life in the United States. But education level is just one factor of a complex picture that Case and Deaton were beginning to paint.

Lack of social support, joblessness, general job insecurity, inequity, and more all began to tell a story of the slippages that had become more and more a part of daily life in America for those with a high school level of education or less. These declines in quality of life are revealed throughout the exploration of various texts about the opioid epidemic. I have chosen to focus upon the opioid overdose portion of deaths of despair because, in part, that portion of deaths have been folded into our cultural and political milieu the most. Deaths related to the opioid epidemic that factor into *deaths of despair* was the reason for the declaration of a public health emergency by the Trump Administration in 2017. Overdose rates climbing in the United States, steadily becoming one of the top reasons for death in the country, merits a study of how it is rhetorically grappled with. The death rates were so alarming and the costs to the country were so high, the nation had to respond and find a novel way to approach this issue. There are also factors that make these deaths easier to discern and to track.

It was the naming, *deaths of despair,* that first brought the opioid epidemic to my attention. Case's observation that these deaths ought to be named thusly sparked the idea that this is a rhetorical situation that deserves to be unpacked. While I do not unpack it entirely, this book is a start in understanding the communication contours and rhetorical dynamics of the opioid epidemic. What Case does by naming it, and that name being widely accepted, is a rhetorical foundation for unpacking the cause, context, and issue as a whole. Star Medzerian Vanguri states, "Names differ from common nouns in that they identify rather than describe; they denote rather than connote. . . .they work to exert new meaning."[5] This also serves as an entry point for my case studies. This book focuses on the rhetorical facets of the opioid epidemic. There are many full-length books that identify various causes of the opioid epidemic, define the issue of the opioid epidemic, and explore possible ways out of the epidemic, but none that explore the rhetoric of the opioid epidemic itself. I will analyze texts from this portion of deaths of despair and find it important to offer a full definition of the term at the outset.

The opioid epidemic is defined by staggering rates of use, overdose, and deaths due to the use of opioids in the United States. According to the National Institute on Drug Abuse (NIDA), "The Centers for Disease Control and Prevention estimates that the total 'economic burden' of prescription opioid misuse alone in the United States is $78.5 billion a year, including the costs of healthcare, lost productivity, addiction treatment, and criminal justice involvement."[6] With an estimated 128 deaths a day, and billions of dollars spent a year, the opioid epidemic is one of the deadliest and most economically costly issues the nation has experienced. It is an epidemic that has taken America by surprise, even though, after looking at several of the contributing factors, it should not be a surprise at all. Rather, it should be more of a foregone conclusion that something as devastating as this on a mass-scale would occur.

A complex web of forces—such as inequity, lack of social support, decline of marriage rates, education being inaccessible by large swaths of the working-class, globalization, massive economy failures in 2008, more

Americans reporting chronic pain starting around the 1970s—lay the groundwork for this uniquely American epidemic. Prescription opioids are a major contributing factor to the epidemic. Elizabeth Finkelman and J. Michael McGinnis have written extensively about the "emergence of the epidemic," and report:

> By the late 1990s, many health care organizations had adopted the mandate that pain must be assessed and treated, and the effectiveness of pain treatment became an important determinant of patient satisfaction scores. A major unintended consequence of this was the overutilization of opioids as the first-line treatment of chronic, non-cancer pain. In conjunction, pharmaceutical companies saw clear opportunities to develop and market new opioid drugs for this purpose, with OxyContin (extended-release oxycodone) being among the most prominent examples.[7]

Overprescribing opioids, misleading marketing from pharmaceutical companies claiming opioid pain killers were nonaddictive and totally safe, and the inclusion of pain as the "fifth vital sign" also fed the opioid epidemic.[8] These factors reshaped the field of medicine and doctor-patient expectations when it came to pain management and treatment. Anna Lembke, a medical doctor and addiction specialist, comments, "The majority of my patients who were misusing prescription drugs were *not* getting their drugs from a drug dealer; they were getting them from a doctor. Sometimes I was the unwitting prescriber."[9] I include this anecdote to demonstrate the ways in which the powerful lobbying of pharmaceutical companies and marketing of opioid-based pain killers were rampant. So much so that even well-meaning and well-trained medical doctors were inadvertently fueling the flames of this epidemic. By 2001, the problem of overprescribing opioid pain killers was out of control and in dire need of intervention.

Though medicine shifted to offer more opioid prescriptions, there was and still exists a distinct lag in how treatment of dependence on these types of drugs should be handled. Furthermore, how the medical field is failing its patients it set up for addiction is also a difficult pill to swallow. A significant component of how the opioid epidemic began is now being held responsible for this problem and is viewed as a central part of the solution. Finkelman and McGinnis assert:

> For those suffering from opioid use disorder, 80% are not receiving treatment. They face formidable treatment barriers not as much from the complexities of addiction treatment as from the reality that the financial, professional, social, and cultural influences at work in our health care system are structured to discourage engagement.[10]

The healthcare system that provided a pathway to addiction is not adequately prepared to assist patients in their recovery from addiction. Few options exist for getting off of prescription pain killers. When prescriptions stopped being doled out so easily, patients who found themselves dependent on opioids had little choice but to turn to heroin and other illegal methods of procurement.[11] Even medically-assisted treatment, or MAT, has many misunderstandings and financial barriers for both providers and patients alike. Many providers do not go through the few extra steps to become qualified to prescribe for medically-assisted treatment, medical settings and clinics that provide that service are far and few between, and there is a daunting stigma that prevents over 80% of patients in need of treatment from seeking it out.[12]

I will quote Case and Deaton's most recent book, *Deaths of Despair and the Future of Capitalism,* at length here to assist with the depiction of whom the opioid epidemic largely impacts directly:

> Our story of deaths of despair; of pain; of addiction, alcoholism, and suicide; of worse jobs with lower wages; of declining marriage; and of declining religion is mostly a story of non-Hispanic white Americans without a four-year degree. In 2018, the Census Bureau estimated that there were 171 million Americans between the ages of twenty-five and sixty-four. Of those, 62 percent were white non-Hispanics, and 62 percent of those did not have a four-year college degree; the less educated white Americans who are the group at risk are 38 percent of the working-age population. The economic forces that are harming labor are common to all working-class Americans, regardless of race or ethnicity, but the stories of blacks and whites are markedly different.[13]

Case and Deaton point to declining rates of marriage and religion, not as normative values, but rather, markers of social support commonly associated with a sense of a collective that can be measured. Other cultural factors, such as individualism and the concept of the American dream—most often an assumed privilege of white Americans—also were identified as stolen away. F. D. Scutchfield and C. William Keck, public health experts, identify a robust individualistic culture in the United States as part of this decline:

> Individuals blame themselves for their changing circumstances and feel desperate and depressed. But the same is true of African Americans and Hispanics, so why have they not experienced this increasing mortality? One can speculate that Whites have a greater expectation that they will have a job, family, and reasonable economic life. African Americans and Hispanics, because of their experience with racism, may not have the same expectations.[14]

Early in their research, race plays a factor in the opioid epidemic. Case and Deaton's findings yield a picture of white, working-class Americans with a high school education or less as the most at-risk.

Disconnection with society and self, either due to lack of social connection or economic struggles, are large drivers of the epidemic. Furthermore, Scutchfield and Keck cite economic struggles as a major factor for why we are seeing the worst of the opioid epidemic currently:

> Income inequality has been expanding in the United States over the past two to three decades, but accelerated during and after the recession of 2008. Globalization and automation have been the main contributors to the loss of low-tech manufacturing jobs and wage stagnation. Workers today with a limited education can no longer be guaranteed well-paying jobs with good benefits, and find themselves in a situation in which they will not fare as well as their parents economically and socially.[15]

Loneliness, isolation, inequity, loss of a sense of self-worth, joblessness and underemployment all contributed to the opioid epidemic and continue to do so. Isolation and loneliness have been found to correlate with rates of reporting physical pain and opioid use.[16] These factors also contribute to an individual's perception of pain and often lead them to doctor's offices to find solutions for their pain with the goal of feeling better.

White Americans being the predominant group impacted has been significant, I contend, to frame the opioid epidemic as a public health matter rather than a criminal and punitive matter. There are several historical and institutional layers that contribute to this. Ashley Ferrell's research on the implementation of comprehensive engagement user sites (or CUES) in Philadelphia to assist with safe heroin injection in the city writes about groups that disrupted the medicalized narrative of the opioid epidemic, "Although the city's framing brought Philadelphia's public health lineage to the forefront, other Philadelphians pointed out that the city's decision to welcome the development of CUES while also adopting and employing the label of 'public health' was just that: a rhetorical choice."[17] Whites in America are a privileged group and are met with less institutional and societal barriers than other demographics.

White Americans typically have better access to healthcare and receive better care in healthcare settings. They are also more likely to be taken at their word when they report pain than nonwhite patients. Ronald Wyatt, M.D., M.H.A, points to a few findings helpful to illustrate the challenges patients face during treatment interactions with medical doctors and clinicians. Wyatt cites, "African Americans and Hispanics were less likely than white patients to receive any pain medication and more likely to receive lower doses of pain medication, despite higher pain scores."[18] The reverse is true for white patients, whom more regularly have their reported pain greeted with seriousness and treatment plans, including the use of opioid pain killers and other nonpharmacological approaches. Wyatt reports, "There is a significant gap between the evaluation and treatment of pain in white people and its evaluation and treatment in African American and Hispanic people."[19] Most medical doctors and clinicians are woefully undertrained and underprepared during their educational process when it comes to pain management and assessment in general.[20] Wyatt points to a few contributing factors to the gap, such as the, "conscious or unconscious negative racial attitudes and stereotyping that affect clinical decision-making despite evidence-based guidelines" as well as poor access to pharmacies and general health literacy as broader social barriers.[21]

A revealing *Washington Post* article titled, *A new divide in American death,* offers a dynamic and moving story about deaths of despair and focuses primarily on the opioid component. Authors Joel Achenbach and Dan Keating explain, "Whites stand out for their high rate of opioid use. Americans represent 5 percent of the world's population but consume at least 80 percent of its prescription opioids. And whites, for complex sociological and economic reasons, are far more likely than blacks or Hispanics to be prescribed opioids."[22] In spite of the population numbers in the United States, our country uses the most prescription opioids in the world and is doing so at an alarming rate. Cultural and societal views in America about pain and the access to these powerful prescription drugs are major contributing factors to the epidemic. Clearly, the problem is multifactored and layered. Case and Deaton argue:

> In the 1970s and 1980s, African Americans working in inner cities experienced events that, in retrospect, share some features with what happened to working-class whites thirty years later. The first wave of globalization hit blacks particularly hard, and jobs in the central city became scarce for this long-disadvantaged group. . . . Crime rates rose, as did morality from violence, from drug overdoses in the crack cocaine epidemic, and from HIV/AIDS, which disproportionately affected blacks. Blacks, always the least favored group, had that status reinforced by being the first to experience the downside of a changing national and global economy that was increasingly shedding less skilled workers.[23]

Whites being the most predominant group impacted certainly plays a role in why the opioid epidemic fairly quickly picked up a public health frame and was viewed more sympathetically. Whereas, given the United States' policies and history of the "war on drugs," African American communities were treated much differently in the worst of crack cocaine use during the mid-1980s and early 1990s. Ferrell's rhetorical investigation of the specific treatment of the opioid epidemic in Philadelphia, the first city to implement CUEs in the whole country, has parts of the community there to remind of the mistreatment of African American communities in the past, "They deliberately interrupted this medicalized narrative by introducing memories of another 'epidemic' of substance use, the 'crack epidemic' of the late 1980s and early 1990s, that disproportionately harmed communities of color and that the city had contradictorily treated as a criminal concern rather than a public health issue."[24] Criminal and deviancy frames were exclusively used during the height of that issue across the nation. Those frames were also used during the height of fear and panic over HIV/AIDS in America around the same time period. The memory of that is not so distant and still resonates, as the example from Ferrell's work reminds us, and is part of why I find the rhetorical study of how the opioid epidemic is treated rhetorically important.

NOTES

1. "Combatting the Overdose Epidemic," *Centers for Disease Control,* March 19, 2020, https://www.cdc.gov/drugoverdose/epidemic/index.html.
2. Anne Case and Angus Deaton, "Mortality and Morbidity in the 21st Century," *Brookings Papers on Economic Activity*, Spring (2017): 400.
3. Ibid, 398.
4. Anne Case and Angus Deaton, *Deaths of Despair and the Future of Capitalism* (New Jersey: Princeton University Press, 2020), 3.
5. Star Medzerian Vanguri, "Toward a Rhetorical Onomastics." In *Rhetorics of Names and Naming,* edited by Star Medzerian Vanguri (New York: Routledge, 2016), 1.
6. "Opioid Overdose Crisis," *National Institute on Drug Abuse,* May 27, 2020, https://www.drugabuse.gov/drug-topics/opioids/opioid-overdose-crisis.
7. Elizabeth M. Finkelman and J. Michael McGinnis, "The Emergence of an Epidemic." In *A Public Health Guide to Ending the Opioid Epidemic*, edited by Jay C. Butler, and Michael R. Fraser (Oxford: Oxford University Press, 2019), 11.
8. Ibid, 11.
9. Anna Lembke, M.D., *Drug Dealer, MD: How Doctors Were Duped, Patients Got Hooked, and Why It's So Hard to Stop* (Baltimore: Johns Hopkins University Press, 2016), 2.
10. Ibid, 14.
11. Nicholas D. Kristof and Sheryl WuDunn, *Tightrope: Americans Reaching for Hope* (New York: Alfred A. Knopf, 2020), 82.
12. Ibid, 15.
13. Anne Case and Angus Deaton, *Deaths of Despair and the Future of Capitalism* (New Jersey: Princeton University Press, 2020), 4.
14. F. D. Scutchfield and C. William Keck, 2017, "Deaths of Despair: Why? What to Do?," *American Journal of Public Health* 107 (10): 1565.
15. Ibid, 1565.

16. Erin Blakemore, "Neuroscientists Think One Way to Fight Opioid Addiction is to Tackle Loneliness," *The Washington Post,* December 1, 2018, https://www.washingtonpost.com/national/health-science/neuroscientist-thinks-one-way-to-fight-opioid-addiction-is-to-tackle-loneliness/2018/11/30/8f651440-f33d-11e8-80d0-f7e1948d55f4_story.html.

17. Ashley P. Ferrell, 2019, "'Righting Past Wrongs': Rhetorical Disidentification and Historical Reference in Response to Philadelphia's Opioid Epidemic," *Rhetoric & Public Affairs* 22 (4): 540–541

18. Ronald Wyatt, M.D., M.H.A., "Pain and Ethnicity," *American Medical Association Journal of Ethics,* May 2013, https://journalofethics.ama-assn.org/article/pain-and-ethnicity/2013-05.

19. Ibid.

20. Anna Lembke, M.D., *Drug Dealer, MD: How Doctors Were Duped, Patients Got Hooked, and Why It's So Hard to Stop* (Baltimore: Johns Hopkins University Press, 2016), 2.

21. Ronald Wyatt, M.D., M.H.A., "Pain and Ethnicity," *American Medical Association Journal of Ethics,* May 2013, https://journalofethics.ama-assn.org/article/pain-and-ethnicity/2013-05.

22. Joel Achenbach and Dan Keating, "A New Divide in American Death," *The Washington Post*, April 10, 2016, online multimedia story, https://www.washingtonpost.com/sf/national/2016/04/10/a-new-divide-in-american-death/?utm_term=.6b948ce6c5e4.

23. Anne Case and Angus Deaton, *Deaths of Despair and the Future of Capitalism* (New Jersey: Princeton University Press, 2020), 5.

24. Ashley P. Ferrell, 2019, "'Righting Past Wrongs': Rhetorical Disidentification and Historical Reference in Response to Philadelphia's Opioid Epidemic," *Rhetoric & Public Affairs* 22 (4): 535.

Chapter 2

Tattered Social Fabric and Dashed Expectations

Documenting the Epidemic through Documentary Films

Mortality rates are on the rise in the United States. Life expectancy is decreasing. At the time I am writing, according to the *Centers for Disease Control,* "two out of three drug overdose deaths involve an opioid." Furthermore, the *Centers for Disease Control* reports, "Overdoses involving opioids killed more than 47,000 people in 2017, and 36% of those deaths involved prescription opioids."[1] With numbers continuing to rise and alarming statistics, visualizing the epidemic in a compelling way seems imperative. Jeffrey Fleishman of the *Los Angeles Times* puts it eloquently, "America's heroin and opioid scourge is intimate and distant, resounding and silent."[2] Perhaps the topic of the opioid epidemic itself is an ineloquent one, which may account for the lag in filmic response. And the lag in response from the Nation as a whole. Even though the signs were there as early as 1998.[3] But looking is difficult. Especially when swaths of the country can avoid looking altogether. Part of the avoidance is long standing due to factors such as race and class impacting how the country responds to drug epidemics. According to Theodore L. Caputi of the *Health Equity Research Laboratory* at Harvard, for too long, our country has:

> stigmatized substance use disorders as a moral failing on the part of the lower classes—poor urban blacks and rural whites—and designed policy focused on preventing crime perpetrated by users rather than helping the users themselves. This largely racist and classist stigma inundated the field, and for too long, too many researchers, clinicians and policymakers were complicit in accepting substance use disorders as a low-class vice rather than a human medical condition.[4]

Documentaries are media that can bring attention to this issue and hopefully help with shifting the general public opinion about substance use disorders. The opioid epidemic is not affecting every tier of society and geographical region in the same way. The white population impacted by the opioid epidemic has brought about attention, resources, and marshaled "medical and political attention" that substance use disorders desperately needed and were not being served properly.[5] Part of this need is due to the long history of stigma and a lack of public support for public health measures. Furthermore, Dr. Caputi argues that through better awareness and infrastructure, "we will be better equipped to address the continued opioid epidemic among whites, the surge of opioid fatalities in the African American community and all future substance use epidemics, regardless of which population is most severely impacted."[6] Understanding the opioid epidemic and the ways it has been shaping approaches to addiction and addiction services is important for understanding the power of the frames used in the way the epidemic is represented through media for the general public. Even though every region has been impacted by 2020, some have been experiencing the epidemic in more deadly ways and for much longer. These two documentaries take a close look at some of the geographical areas most impacted by the epidemic.

Documentary films, particularly during an age of dwindling budgets for investigative journalism, have been a productive outlet for revealing information about the opioid epidemic. Bloomfied and Sangalang cite the power of documentaries to disseminate information about health to the general public, "Health issues are also being addressed in the realm of entertainment. Documentary films in particular (i.e., *Food, Inc., Killer at Large,* and *Food Fight)* are an accessible source of health information for the public" (Nisbet & Aufderheide, 2009).[7] The opioid epidemic has been part of the push for seeing substance use disorders as medical conditions. Documentaries, seen as an accessible source for health information, are part of changing that vision. Around 2017, alongside the deadliest year for the opioid epidemic being driven by an increase in fentanyl and other synthetic opioid-related deaths, a "surge" of documentaries began to surface that took the opioid epidemic on.[8] Fleishman remarks that Elaine McMillion Sheldon's documentary is one of the "most unflinching and disturbing portraits of a numbing and perilous terrain."[9] Documentaries, such as McMillion Sheldon's *Heroin(e)* and Mark Levin's *One Nation Under Stress: Deaths of Despair in the United States,* are apt and compelling documentary films. McMillion Sheldon focuses on her home state of West Virginia. Levin's prior work on documentaries about socioeconomic inequities in the United States positioned him well to take a look at inequities and issues of health.

The dynamics and nuances of the epidemic present complicated pictures. There are no easy answers. Identifying underlying causes is a complicated venture. Identifying solutions is just as daunting. Capturing it for an audience is even more complicated. Yet, these documentaries have garnered success and attention for their vision. Particularly McMillion Sheldon's *Heroin(e),* which was nominated for best-documentary-short Oscar. McMillion Sheldon is also an Emmy and Peabody award-winner. Mark Levin, critically acclaimed independent filmmaker and fellow Peabody award-winner, teamed up with *CNN*'s Emmy award-winning chief medical correspondent Dr. Sanjay Gupta to make *One Nation Under Stress: Deaths of Despair in the United States* (*One Nation Under Stress* hereafter). Dr. Gupta guides the audience through some of the hardest hit places in the country in a narrative meets verité style documentary. Each focus on individual cases in order to craft a compelling portrait of the opioid epidemic that the White House declared a "public health emergency" in October 2017.[10] Both feature an intimate look into what the epidemic *looks* like and instruct what the epidemic also *feels* like for those battling it.

In what follows, I closely examine scenes featuring the professional expert guides and the experiential experts whose lives are transformed in each documentary. I argue the narrative arc of individuals afflicted does important rhetorical work in order to compel the audience to take the perspective of the professional expert guides. Both documentaries share the thread of identifying the underlying cause of the epidemic. Each also recommends compassionate, medical, and behavioral efforts to turn the tide of the epidemic. *Heroin(e)* emphasizes the solution while *One Nation Under Stress* emphasizes the underlying causes of the epidemic. Each articulate their main points through the narrative arc of those suffering through the perspective of a professional medical expert. Through potent synecdoches—Mickey Watson and Jan Rader in *Heroin(e)* and Angela Glass and Dr. Sanjay Gupta in *One Nation Under Stress*—provide audiences an *intimate* and *resounding* portrait of the opioid epidemic. Each synecdoche draw attention to the tensions and potential perceptions about epidemic, which will be explored in the analysis.

I demonstrate how a public health frame and medicalization are achieved through synecdochal rhetoric throughout the documentaries by presenting the information from the perspective of public health officials, affirms the epidemic as a disease rather than a moral failing of individuals who are addicts. I identify how the public health frame and medicalization of the issue are visually, textually, and verbally asserted as well. Experts from both medical and first responder professions, a doctor and fire chief, guide the audience and instruct what the epidemic looks and feels like. *Experts* include what I identify as professional experts and experiential experts. Professional experts are guides for the audience and are those in the documentaries whose profession is to medically assist those afflicted. The experiential experts are the afflicted individuals, whose testimony and personal accounts, expand upon the knowledge that can assist with stymieing the tide of the epidemic that has swept the country. These individuals serve as powerful synecdoches that shape the rhetoric of the epidemic.

A BRIEF LITERATURE REVIEW OF DOCUMENTARY FILM

Documentaries invite us to "share its meanings" and guide the viewer to identify with the politics of a social issue, election season, and more.[11] Thomas Benson remarks that documentaries develop a compelling rhetoric of "sentimental identification," wherein the audience is invited to take on the meanings shared by those featured on the screen.[12] Identification is essential to the rhetorical work of documentaries. The visual and aural components of a documentary function simultaneously as argument and evidence. Thomas Rosteck and Thomas S. Frentz state, "At the heart of the documentary enterprise is the technological capacity to record a visual and aural record of a particular piece of the world, a recording that comprises the evidentiary quality of the documentary account."[13] This process is described by Nichols as a "classic alternation between appeals to evidence and appeals to audience" and powerfully "couple[s] evidence *and* emotion."[14] The medium itself rhetorically assists by putting visual and aural tropes in front of the audience.

The audience is effectively witnessing the testimony of those on the front lines as they recount their lived experience. The medium of documentary enables the audience to see the opioid epidemic with their own eyes as they are guided through it from both sides: the professional expert and the experiential expert testimonies and accounts. Bradford Vivian remarks of "the sensuousness of a given medium" that "involves consumers of mass culture in a liminal time that approximates the fundamentally riven—indeed, untimely—temporal experience of witnesses to historical tragedy, trauma, and violence."[15] Emotion, evidence, and guides to identify with through these visits into the overwhelming epidemic are at the center of my close reading of the documentaries. Carl Plantinga remarks, "Emotions can also be used for rhetorical purposes. People routinely turn to their feelings for guidance when making judgments and decisions."[16] Each documentary demonstrates a compassionate emotional response through professional experts the audience can comfortably identify with: a fire chief and a medical doctor. Their compassionate response becomes the model for the viewer. Their emotions, as they guide the viewer through the tumult of the epidemic, are the ones the audience is invited to share in, make judgements, and decisions about the epidemic.

The filmmakers are building a particular case about the opioid epidemic: identifying an underlying cause and bearing out the fruit of compassionate treatment approaches through successful narrative arcs of conversion. Testimony from experts, both professional experts and experiential experts, directly impacted by the issue is a powerful way to reinforce these arguments. Bill Nichols speaks of the powerful ability of the documentary interview that "generates *testimony* about the characterological dimensions of this social performance, or life."[17] Witnessing, from those who testify as to the nature of the epidemic and possible solutions, is another key function of these documentaries that are affectively conveying the trauma of individuals. Therefore, the trauma of the entire country as well. Barbie Zelizer states, "bearing witness moves individuals from the personal act of 'seeing' to the adoption of a public stance by which they become part of a collective working through trauma together."[18] Zelizer's work around photographs translates to the role of documentary with regard to mediating trauma, moving toward recovery, and "help return the collective to its pre-traumatic unified state."[19] This transition from "seeing" to the "adoption of a public stance" is critical work the documentaries take on unabashedly. Testimony is a powerful rhetorical vehicle. Witnessing the epidemic is key for identification as well as action, or support for action, that can be voted for and carried about by public health officials and first responders.

Furthermore, the individual testimony featured simultaneously represents a specific and a broad view of the epidemic. The epidemic impacts the entire country and the documentaries propose the individual experiences featured can and should be extrapolated to the rest of the country. Rosteck and Frentz point to the power of the documentary film to induce "a simultaneous particularizing and universalizing symbolic movement" for the viewer.[20] Kenneth Burke describes the synecdoche as a representation—"part for the whole" or a "microcosm"—which enables identification and the perception of material realities.[21] The reduction of the whole epidemic to parts, represented in the documentaries, is expanded cognitively out to the whole of the nation by the viewer. I will also show where the professional experts guiding the viewer in each documentary make this relationship, part for whole, explicit. This is essential rhetorical work for representing an epidemic that Nicholas Kristof and Sheryl WuDunn emphasize is "not one town's problem, but a crisis in the American system."[22] Tackling the entire problem would be too much for the documentary as well as the cognition of the viewer. Synecdoche rhetorically reduces the whole of the epidemic to a consumable and compelling portion for the audience.

Effectively reducing the epidemic down to a representative part for whole in a compelling way is part of the work the documentaries are up to. Rosteck and Frentz find "the trope of synecdoche is perfectly suited to describe the persuasive dimensions and rhetorical action of many documentaries. For it seems that it is via the cognitive operations described by synecdoche that the documentary magnifies the specific case while enacting the universal within the concrete through the layering of the conventions of narrative over it."[23] The narratives focus upon individuals, offer up specific cases, and then extrapolate to the whole nation what the compassionate, medical responses ought to be to this devastating epidemic as well as what the underlying causes are.

SUMMARIES OF DOCUMENTARIES

Critically-acclaimed director Elaine McMillion Sheldon takes a deep look at her own home state of West Virginia in the Oscar nominated *Heroin(e).* The focus of the concise, thirty-nine-minute documentary is the heart of the epidemic: compassionate treatment and outreach. It is described on *Netflix's* site as a documentary that "shows how the chain of compassion holds one town together."[24] *Heroin(e)* follows three women: Jan Rader, Deputy Chief Fire Department, Judge Patricia Keller of Cabell County, and Necia Freeman, of the Brownbag Ministry. Each is directly assisting sufferers of the opioid epidemic in Huntington-Cabell County, West Virginia. Jan Rader takes the helm of the individual the audience spends the most time with and, therefore, will be a focus of my analysis.

In *One Nation Under Stress*, the audience follows Dr. Sanjay Gupta as he interviews experts on the issue of deaths of despair. Experts include medical doctors, researchers from various academic backgrounds, those suffering from opioid addiction themselves, and those who have lost loved ones to deaths of despair. Dr. Gupta ventures to some of the hardest hit regions in the United States of the opioid epidemic, including portions of the Rust Belt in Pennsylvania and Michigan, as well as a small town in Texas.

Both documentaries dive deep into the human portrait that is the opioid epidemic, of which deaths of despair are part and parcel. The audience follows the action of the epidemic in an "on the ground" meets verité perspective. Each focus upon those whom directly interact with those afflicted in powerful ways. *One Nation Under Stress* focuses more upon the underlying causes of deaths of despair in general, with a focus on the opioid epidemic. *Heroin(e)* focuses on the opioid epidemic and the direct efforts to save lives and stymie the epidemic progress in their small town. Gupta and Rader guide the audience through the devastating, daunting, and downright overwhelming facets of the epidemic. I have included a documentary with a focus on underlying causes, *One Nation Under Stress,* and a documentary with the focus of treatment, *Heroin(e),* to garner a broader view of the discourses of deaths of despair. Holding them next to one another will also enrich what can be learned about the rhetoric in the medium of documentary tackling the challenge of an epidemic that is, according to the Centers for Disease Control and Prevention, claiming the lives of 130 Americans each day.[26]

CONCERN TO HOPE: NARRATIVE CONVERSIONS

Heroin(e) and *One Nation Under Stress* both represent the epidemic gripping the United States through individual's stories. Each documentary provides individual accounts from parts of the country that have been most impacted, and for the longest since the beginning of the era of deaths of despair began in 1999, to represent the whole of the epidemic. Synecdochic stories offer a simultaneous feeling of concern and hope for the nation. I analyze the conversion of Mickey Watson in *Heroin(e)* and Angela Glass in *One Nation Under Stress.*

On the medical profession's side of the epidemic, Rader serves as the narrative conversion arc in *Heroin(e).* While not a sufferer of despair, Rader directly serves and saves those afflicted in her community. Her career has been defined by the epidemic in many ways. Rader is the guide in *Heroin(e)* for the audience. She serves as a comfortable person the audience can identify with. It is through her eyes and her transformation over the course of the documentary the audience comes to understand the epidemic through. Over scenes of the small town of Huntington, Rader's voiceover describes the problem. She explains the underlying causes of the epidemic, "West Virginia is mainly a blue-collar state in general. So, we have a lot of people who work hard for a living. Do a lot of physical labor. There's a lot of injuries. A lot of people in this area got hooked on pills through a legitimate injury and now have moved onto heroin because they can't get pills anymore." The medical frame, through a first responder as an expert operating in a place well-versed with the epidemic, is firmly set within the first few minutes of the documentary. Rader's compassionate approach is at the heart of the documentary.

Within two minutes of the opening scene, the audience sees an overdose reversal and the survivor being transported by ambulance. While riding along with Rader as she shows the audience houses where people have not been rescued from overdose, white text appears on the screen over the depressed looking neighborhoods of Huntington that reads, "Huntington, West Virginia has been called the overdose capital of America." Mickey, who is first encountered around the midpoint of the film, is contrasted to these early visions of the epidemic. Mickey's narrative arc serves as a demonstration of hope and evidence of Rader's efforts being effective and worthwhile.

Bridging the gap between the specific case to the universal is a rhetorical maneuver seen explicitly while the audience is riding along to the local hospital after responding to an overdose call. *Heroin(e)* demonstrates how this particular case of West Virginia is endemic of the epidemic as a whole. Rader bridges the gap between the particular and the universal when she states:

> You know, I see this as a countrywide problem that has the potential to bankrupt the country. You know we conservatively estimated that Cabell County, that's about 96,000 people, spent about one-hundred million dollars in healthcare costs associated with I.V. drug use in 2015. That's one small county, in one small state. I don't—I cannot even fathom what it's gonna look like when it plateaus. But I know it will be welcomed.[27]

Cabell County is a synecdoche for the greater whole of the epidemic. By understanding the cost of life and money to one county, the viewer can then extrapolate outward to imagine and better comprehend the trillions of the dollars and thousands of lives lost. Just seeing the numbers is not as effective as this potent synecdoche.

As a dispenser of the overdose reversal drug Naloxone, coordinator for its dispersal to first responders, and active advocate for nuanced recovery efforts, Rader's conversion work is consistently demonstrated through those she saves in the documentary. The audience rides along with her during a typical day of work. Rader directly contributes to the conversion of sufferers to survivors. Mickey comes into focus as a model of what success looks like in a hard-hit part of the country. The audience sees the transformation possible with a compassionate approach to the epidemic that focuses on the medical and behavioral health frames of the issue. Mickey, a local in the small town where Rader works, is contrasted to calls responded to for overdose reversal in the first half of the documentary. Mickey is the synecdoche. His story of recovery is also the bedrock of Rader's transformation that we witness in *Heroin(e).*

MICKEY WATSON

The segment with Mickey Watson demonstrates the oscillation between various types of information throughout the documentary well. Personal accounts from both sides of the epidemic as well as hard facts and data are both present to round out the picture of the epidemic. The statistics are personified through success stories. The first success story featured is that of Mickey Watson. He is introduced after a long lead up through Rader's account and interactions with other county and city officials. Data and facts about Rader's medical approach are supported with an individual who personifies what Rader testifies to in a public safety meeting. The audience can literally see with their own eyes the proof of Rader's approach being effective.

Mickey's segment has a fairly long lead up in the documentary. It opens with scenic, wide shots of a train passing by a body of water in the town. Then it cuts to a hand-held camera close-up shot of Rader seated in the audience at the meeting. At a Cabell-Huntington County Health Department Public Safety meeting, the audience follows Rader through her interactions with others in the community whom are on what I refer to as the professional side of the opioid epidemic. By that I mean it is their profession or part of their job to assist those afflicted. Law enforcement is updating various county officials in attendance about recent statistics for non-fatal overdose, which have risen over the last year. The voice of Scott Lemley, Criminal Intelligence Analyst, Huntington Police Department is out of frame so the audience can hear the statistics, but identify with Rader's reactions to them. She shakes her head and says, "geez," when he announces that non-fatal overdoses are up in the city of Huntington. The camera angle then cuts to a wide shot of Lemley as he emphasizes "the shift from pills to heroin" as he stands at a podium at the front of the conference room with a chart revealing data about types of fentanyl.[28] Lemley explains further, "now we are seeing another shift, from pills to fentanyl, to stuff that's even more stronger," and the camera cuts back to the close-up of Rader making notes on a pad in front of her. For much of the audience, they may not be aware of the facts and details of the opioid epidemic. The audience is processing the information along with Rader and reading her responses as the ones they should emulate as their own.

The statistics are alarming for her small town. This makes the synecdoche all that more powerful. If one small town is having this large of an issue, it makes it easier to extrapolate outward from there that the rest of the nation is struggling as well. Rader has already articulated to the audience that what is happening in Huntington can be extrapolated out to the rest of the country in an earlier scene. According to the National Institute on Drug Abuse (NIDA), "The Centers for Disease Control and Prevention estimates that the total 'economic burden' of prescription opioid misuse alone in the United States is $78.5 billion a year."[29] The audience in the room shares in the revelation that there are drugs even stronger than pain pills and heroin. Furthermore, that fentanyl is driving the epidemic statistics even higher. This information is received by those in the room with discomfort. People can be seen visibly shifting in their chairs. The shot cuts from the medium shot of Lemley presenting back to the close-up of Rader as she stands from her chair and interrupts, "I just want to say that those figures could be a lot worse, especially the deaths, if it hadn't been for this health department." This is an incredibly powerful scene. It works in a few ways. First, the audience whom is already comfortable with Rader, is beginning to see the raw numbers and more detailed information regarding the epidemic in Huntington. The first half of the documentary focuses upon individuals being saved by Naloxone by Rader and her brigade of fire fighters. The viewer follows Rader on calls responding to overdoses and interacting with officials on a one-on-one or small group setting regarding Naloxone. Now the emphasis on overdose reversal and distributing Naloxone effectively is viewed in a broader, more data-driven setting. This really drives the point home for the audience about the need for Naloxone and Rader's unending compassion.

While bridging the gap between the particular to universal even more, the audience is also introduced to an oppositional argument to the distribution and use of Naloxone. Since this is something that the audience may encounter in the real world, it is an effective portion of the meeting to include. Rader reassures the group that Naloxone is not "enabling" opioid use and her explanation, naturally occurring in the meeting, effectively acts to inform the audience along with her peers. It also gives an opportunity to describe further what Naloxone does to the person's system in the state of overdose. Rader explains, "Most people actually get mad because you've thrown them into withdrawal." This counters the misperception that Naloxone will, as the other official states he has heard around town that access to Naloxone is "empowering the addicts," and thereby presents another perspective the audience may have also encountered before viewing the documentary. The member of the officials offers a counterargument that Rader can demonstrate as false immediately and the audience can adopt that information.

Next, the long lead up to Mickey shifts to seeing how Rader's efforts have worked through a potent synecdoche. The audience ventures along to another scene that features Mickey himself. The audience is about to see with their own eyes the power of saving those in overdose with Naloxone and medical recovery. Before leaving the meeting, the audience hears Rader's passionate testimony for the medical approach and then will visually see she was referring to Mickey:

> The only qualification for getting into long term recovery, is that you have to be alive. And I don't care if I save somebody 50 times. That's 50 chances to get into long term recovery. People do go into long term recovery. And they do, um, become productive citizens. Tax paying citizens. And they are going to, in turn, help more and more people suffering from addiction. So, uh, I truly believe that even though we have this doom and gloom, thank you Debbie Downer, that I think we certainly need to focus on the successes that we as a community have had.

The scene cuts from Rader's moving testimony to wide shot of a neighborhood. Then to a close-up of art hanging on the wall inside of a modest home. The handheld camera becomes apparent again as a man appears in view in the residence. The intertitle in the lower left corner reads "MICKEY WATSON

Recovering Addict" as he prepares a backpack by his door. A man's voice is heard over the scene of Mickey getting ready to leave, "Last time Jan brought me back, that shit ain't heroin anymore. It's fentanyl and elephant tranquilizer." The handheld camera follows him as he exists the residence. He has long hair. Is wearing a baggy sweatshirt and places a beanie over his head. The voiceover continues, "In the past month, there's been ten people that I know of die." The camera cuts to a close-up of Mickey seated at a café table when he says "But for some damn reason, I'm still sittin' here." The scene cuts to a close-up from behind Mickey as Rader takes him into an excited embrace. The quick cut to an action shot of Rader embracing Mickey implies that it was Rader who saved Mickey. She *is* the reason he is still alive. The question he wonders about in the café is answered in the next scene. He is one of those successes she references in the meeting. One of those she has saved over and over again until he could enter recovery.

Mickey's conversion is not just about himself. He has reached a point to where he demonstrates the next phase of Rader's account to the public safety officials. Rader articulates in that earlier scene in the meeting, right before the audience meets Mickey, that people enter recovery and then "in turn, help more and more people suffering from addiction." What follows builds on the visual argument that Rader's compassion and medical approach works. The camera follows Mickey and Rader as he is showing Rader his current efforts. Mickey and a group of recovering addicts walk the river bank where he used to live while in the thralls of opioid abuse disorder. Mickey and his group are offering supplies, help, and encouragement to people still addicted to enter recovery. Within the first few minutes after the audience sees Rader testify to her peers about Naloxone and nuanced recovery efforts, the audience gets the visual evidence of her efforts working. An exchange between the two solidifies and make certain the conversion of Mickey is articulated is witnessed by the audience. A close-up of Rader telling Mickey about the overdose numbers in the city alternates with close-ups of Mickey's responses.

Rader: We still don't have the numbers yet.

Mickey: Yeah, that's what the papers was saying.

Rader: For 2016's. It's gonna be probably over 80.

Mickey: Deaths?

Rader: (nods)

MICKEY: WAS THAT HIGHER THAN 2015?

> Rader: 2015 was 70 in the county. It's gonna be higher.
>
> Mickey: You know last year's the first year I haven't been a part of that number.
>
> Rader: Yeah, right. I never thought about it that way.
>
> Mickey: I didn't either until you was sitting talking about it. And I was just sitting here thinking, since I lived in Huntington, there hasn't been a year gone by I haven't been a part of the overdose number.
>
> Rader: Wow.

The rapport that Rader has with Mickey—and vice-a-versa—is palpable. They appear to be friends, in spite of how they met. Their friendship is a synecdochal representation of how this public health and medicalization approach can help elsewhere. Compassion is the key to turning this epidemic around. This touching exchange and the compassion from Rader is apparent in these scenes with Mickey. The audience, through their identification with Rader, can feel along with her emotional responses to knowing that Mickey is clean, safe, and is helping others. The compassionate approach to the epidemic is working. Mickey is a synecdoche of success that could be modeled and replicated throughout the country. By identifying with either of these individuals, the viewer can adopt their framing of the issue more easily and begin to change their perceptions or affirm their positive perspective of the epidemic and those suffering.

Rader undergoes an historical transformation herself. At the beginning of the documentary, Rader's intertitle is Deputy Chief. By the end, it is fire chief. An intertitle marks the historical transformation in text across the screen. Marking in words the importance for the audience. Mickey is part of that journey and transformation. Toward the end of the documentary, the audience gets to follow Rader to her swearing in ceremony. She is the first female fire chief in West Virginia history. It is assumed that, in part, her success is due to the way she has progressively taken the helm of changing the epidemic's impact in her county. The audience sees behind the scenes as Rader gets dressed for a press interview and ceremony. She remarks as the audience sees her tying a tie in the mirror, "I suck at ties, just so you know." She smiles a bit. The segment shifts to Rader getting out of her fire vehicle, the red SUV the audience has been riding along with her in, in front of a county building. Over the shoulder and through the viewer of news camera, the audience hears the reporter just out of frame speaking to Rader about her exemplary career and asking her what has prepared her for this new leadership role. Rader remarks, "This is a uh very personally satisfying profession. I can walk away every day thinking or knowing that I made a difference." Cuts to a close-up shot of her and Judge Keller. It cuts to more press inside of the auditorium where the ceremony is being held. A close-up of a woman interviewing Mickey, who has a short haircut and appears more professionally dressed, asks him his reason for coming out to the ceremony. Mickey responds, without missing a beat, "Well, she's the reason why I am sittin' here." He pauses as tears well up in his eyes. "She saved my life twice in a week. It ain't just a job for her. She cares." Rader is shown on stage with Judge Kellner and a few other public officials.

The wide shot of the whole stage cuts to a close-up of Rader approaching the podium. After being sworn in, Rader begins her speech:

> Even though Huntington is experiencing difficult financial issues and an unprecedented public health epidemic, working together, I have no doubt that we will emerge better and stronger as a city and as a community. Today we stand together, proving that anything is possible. The road may be rough with many barricades. Yet, we are all capable of finding the strength within to reach our goals. Thank you all for coming here. And a special thanks to somebody who completely changed my life. More than they will ever know. Mickey.

The medium shot, a view that someone would have while seated in the crowd, zooms when Rader starts with "thank you all for coming here." The zoomed close-up captures her face begin to change. She starts to cry a bit as she talks about Mickey changing her life. The shot cuts to a long shot with Mickey in the center. He is starting to cry as well and looks straight into the camera briefly. A few people start to clap and deliver a standing ovation for Rader. The shot cuts to a close-up, over the shoulder of Rader as her and Mickey embrace. Mickey says, "I love you, Jan." Her face pressed against his, Rader says, "I love you too, honey. I love you too. I'll always be there for you." They end their embrace and the camera pulls back slightly to a medium shot, framing Mickey and Rader, with light streaming in from the doors behind them. Mickey tells her, "If you can get them to care a quarter of what you do, it would change this city." Rader replies, "Absolutely. And that's what we're gonna do." The synecdoche comes in again with this final note of transformation. Rader is in an even more influential position as fire chief and has allies who she has contributed to transforming from afflicted to being on her side of the cause: saving lives.

This final scene with Mickey serves as emotionally compelling, visual evidence for the audience that a compassionate, medical and behavioral health approach works to combat the opioid epidemic. It puts the afflicted and first responders on the same side: opposite the epidemic. Fighting to save lives and change a city. If one of the hardest hit places in the country can do it, the audience can conclude, so can the rest of the country. Rader is the first person the audience sees and rides along with. She begins by showing houses in Huntington where people have died from overdoses. Rader articulates the underlying causes to the epidemic that plagues her small town, "When you add hopelessness and unemployment. And lack of education on top of all that, it's kind of like a recipe for disaster." The transformation to hope at the end of the documentary is potent, yet tempered. The final scene fades to black as the audience departs, the sound of sirens starting up blasts, and Rader responds to yet another overdose call. Our heroine, once again, returns to the fray.

ANGELA GLASS

Angela Glass from Victoria, Texas, offers an arc of concern to hope in *One Nation Under Stress.* Angela's narrative conversion makes the epidemic, while daunting, seem like a worthy effort to take part in order to stymie the tide of devastation the opioid epidemic has wrought. Angela also serves as the shining example of what opioid abuse disorder looks like from a sympathetic perspective with a firm medical frame in place. Her conversion is witnessed by a physician. Dr. Gupta's voiceover explains that Angel's addiction began after becoming dependent upon prescribed opioids after the loss of a child during a difficult pregnancy. The many layers of her suffering, of her despair, summarize the whole of the opioid epidemic in a single individual.

Angela is the first sufferer that Dr. Gupta visits with in the film. She is also the first interview in the documentary that is not the voice and perspective from a professional expert. Angela straddles the line of professional expert and expert in the sense that she is in the thralls of the epidemic. As a nurse, she has medical expertise. As a sufferer, she has expertise based on the experience of becoming addicted to pain pills due to overwhelming stress. She appears three times in the documentary: the beginning, middle, and the end. Angela's transformation punctuates the documentary in a powerful way. The audience follows her conversion from despair to hope as they are learning, from professional experts all about the underlying causes of the epidemic, and come through at the end with Angela in recovery. Like Mickey, her conversion is witnessed by a professional expert and the audience is invited to view the transformation through their eyes. In this case, with Angela, the audience views her conversion arc through Dr. Gupta's eyes and narration.

The scene cuts from first responders out on calls in Angela's town to a medium shot of Angela seated outside. This juxtaposition shows that Angela is close to meeting a similar fate. Her intertitle introduces her to the audience as Dr. Gupta's voice is heard from off camera inquiring, "What does stress look like?" The camera cuts to a close-up of Angela's face as she says, "Stress is ugly." She elaborates that it can cause a variety of problems and looks exhausted as she describes stress. The scene cuts to scenes of Angela interacting with her children and husband in their home. Dr. Gupta's voice narrates over the scene, "In Victoria, Texas, I met Angela. She's a mother. She's a wife. And she's a nurse. And she's being prescribed a huge cocktail of meds for her stress." Scenes showing Angela in her home cut to a picture on screen of her and her family at a gravesite. Angela lost her second child when she was full-term and turned to pills to cope with her stress. Scenes reveal her shifting through prescription pill bottles and taking a fist full of pills in her kitchen. Cutting back to the close-up shot of Angela seated outside, she shares that she is suicidal and thinks about taking all of her hydrocodone and Xanax to "just go to sleep." She starts to tear up and the scene cuts to establishing shots of Victoria and then to an extreme close-up of Dr. Gupta's eyes as he is driving through the streets of Victoria. His voiceover states, "Its hard to hear. And to think that so many Americans have been led down this path of drug dependence." He connects Angela's account to the underlying cause of the epidemic: stress coupled with the desire to "medicate it away." Prescribers and patients alike feed into the problem.

Half way through the documentary, Dr. Gupta checks back in from *CNN* headquarters from afar with Angela as she checks into rehab. The camera cuts from a close-up of Dr. Gupta's eyes watching footage of Angela on screens to a medium shot of Angela in her living room. She explains to the audience, "If I knew I was gonna be here right now, I wouldn't have started taking medication. I don't wish this on anybody." She looks destitute and depressed. The scene cuts to her husband being interviewed. He expresses his support and dedication to Angela and states plainly looking into the camera, "There's only one way to go from here and that's going up." It cuts to them in their truck as he takes Angela to rehab. The audience can see Angela writing out a list in the truck as the camera looks over her shoulder. Her voice narrates the scene and rationale for her transition to rehab, "I want to learn how to cope, other than medicating. That's something that I haven't learned before." The audience is seeing part of her transition. When Dr. Gupta sat down with her in the beginning of the documentary, Angela was considering suicide. Now, with the support of her spouse and family, she enters rehab to learn to move away from medicating with opioids and anti-anxiety pills. The camera follows the couple to rehab and looks through a glass door as they check Angela in. It cuts to the front of the rehab center at dusk.

Dr. Gupta's voice is heard off-camera over the moving scene explaining, "As a doctor, I'm pretty used to knowing the prognosis for my patients. And as I sit here and watch Angela, I don't know how she's going to do. And I don't know what the prognosis is for this epidemic of self-destructive behavior." The scene cuts away from the rehab center to a close-up of Dr. Gupta's eyes as he is watching the rehab scene unfold on screens back at *CNN* headquarters. It cuts to him passing through the hall and the camera stops on a large cardboard cutout of Anthony Bourdain who committed suicide in 2018. Here, the synecdoche of Angela's prognosis representing the prognosis for the entire epidemic is asserted subtly yet, explicitly implies the whole nation's prognosis is uncertain as well. Dr. Gupta himself, as a medical doctor, serves as a medicalization and public health frame throughout the documentary. The close-up of Bourdain is a stark reminder of what is at stake in the deaths of despair of America. The level of seriousness of the epidemic is undeniable and has numerous victims from the realm of popular culture that the audience has heard of and will recognize. Bourdain is one that hits close to the *CNN* family. Bourdain is a synecdoche for broader picture of deaths of despair. Sometimes a celebrity synecdoche can more quickly foster compassion and understanding of a difficult subject. The inclusion of that moment is surely a rhetorical strategy to assist with identification for compassion.

In the last third of the documentary, Dr. Gupta visits Victoria, Texas, again to see how Angela is doing. A year has passed since they first visited. The scene cuts to a close-up of the City of Victoria sign and then to a wide-shot of Dr. Gupta and Angela walking around a small-town downtown. His voiceover narrates the visit and establishes the timeline for how long it had been since he first met with her. Angela looks vibrant. Her hair and makeup are done. She is wearing nice-fitting clothes and has shed her baggy t-shirts and sweats. The scene cuts to a close-up of her smiling into the camera as Dr. Gupta's voice is heard saying, "I couldn't believe what I saw." The transformation is remarkable visually. Angela is smiling and looks alive. The transformation from where Angela was a year ago is a compelling synecdoche. The scene stays on the close-up of Angela as Dr. Gupta's voice can be heard over the shot, "How are you doing?" Off camera Angela can be heard, "I'm doing wonderful." It then cuts to a close-up of Dr. Gupta's face as inquires further, "Are you off all the . . ." Angela interrupts his question, "I'm off everything. I don't take anything at all." The camera cuts to a medium shot of Angela as she responds, "I feel like the medication alters your mind. It alters the way you think." She is testifying to the way in which opioids and anti-anxiety medications transformed her to who she was when she first encounters the audience. Now, the Angela sitting before Dr. Gupta is well, off of all medications, and has gained important coping skills from rehab to deal with her despair. The audience is viewing this transformation through a doctor's perspective and sees her as a patient who has recovered from a disease and her despair simultaneously.

Their conversation clinches this conclusion when Dr. Gupta explains, "I mean, the story typically is as you know tens of thousands of people die every year from these overdoses. But you came out the other side." What Angela asserts next fits into the larger lesson about tattered social fabric and lack of support being underlying causes of the epidemic. Angela explains, "I feel like if there were a lot more people like my husband and my mom and how supportive they were that a lot of people would get help earlier." Care and compassion are consistently pointed to throughout the documentary as ways to combat the underlying causes of the epidemic. Dr. Gupta remarks that "too often we've lost that care and compassion for the larger American family" as the scene transitions to Dr. Gupta visiting another professional expert about the underlying causes of the epidemic. Angela's transformation demonstrates the key points of the documentary in a few ways. First, Angela is met when she is at her lowest. Suffering from opioid abuse disorder and considering suicide, Dr. Gupta talks to Angela about what lead up to that point. The audience sees how this could happen through the vantage point of a medical doctor who is caring and compassionate. Next, Angela does the hard work of going to rehab and letting those who love her support her through her transition away from medicating her despair. Finally, Angela is a vibrant and productive person again who wants to share her story about recovery through her testimony and transformation in the documentary.

RENDERING THE EPIDEMIC VISIBLE

Frenetic camera movement propels the viewer through the opioid epidemic along with the guides. The movement operates to demonstrate and provide evidence simultaneously. The audience connects and identifies with a single individual, Sanjay Gupta in *One Nation Under Stress,* and Jan Rader in *Heroin(e),* by virtue of their expertise. By moving through the epidemic alongside these professional experts, the audience is seeing things through a medical frame. Movement assists with compelling the audience to identify with that frame. The frenetic movement builds on the authenticity of the experience the documentaries build. Plantinga states, "the moving camera, under certain conditions, is like a stand-in for the human body as it moves through the scene."[30] By riding along with Rader and Gupta, the audience takes on their perspective—visually, rationally, and emotionally—as they witness the conversion arcs of experiential experts. Both Rader and Gupta explore the underlying causes and ways to approach the epidemic. Their experiences and view from the front lines of the epidemic become the audience's way of seeing as well as experiencing.

The medicalization and public health frame is enhanced through this frenetic movement. In *Heroin(e),* Rader's perpetual compassion and insistence on the medical and mental health approach is demonstrated with each overdose call she responds to. With the audience running up to an overdose call right on the heels of Rader, she is informed that the house she is entering holds an individual who had already overdosed that same week. The camera bounds up the stairs behind Rader and zooms in on her feet. It visually argues the audience literally "walk in the shoes" of Rader. The next scene zooms in on the action of Rader's life-saving procedures and alternates to close-ups of her face. After the individual responds to a dose of Naloxone, Rader asks, "Cody, have you tried to get clean or anything, honey?" The young man replies that he will check into rehab shortly. Rader affirms him by saying, "Cody, I am really happy to hear that. That is really good." The solution for this individual is a hospital visit and then drug rehabilitation.

In this short scene, the audience witnesses an overdose reversal with Naloxone and the solution, more permanently, is to get the individual to rehabilitation. Not jail. Even though it is the second overdose for that individual in one week, Rader's commitment and compassion stands unwavering. This implies that the audience should adopt that frame for the epidemic as well. The medical frame is affirmed through Rader's response. First, Rader rescues him with the overdose reversal drug. Second, she confirms he is going to a medical and behavioral treatment facility for rehabilitation. This scene reifies and reiterates the scene in an earlier segment in which Rader remarks, "I don't care if I save somebody 50 times. That's 50 chances to get into long term recovery." Just as the narrative arc of Mickey demonstrates, long-term recovery and medical interventions are the solution. Compassion will see the nation through the epidemic.

In *One Nation Under Stress,* the audience is encouraged at every moment to view the epidemic through the perspective of a medical doctor. Following a well-known medical doctor as he travels the country really drives the point home. The medical profession is not presented as entirely clean in this documentary. In an early scene, the audience sits in on a conversation about changes in medicine that drove the opioid epidemic to where it is in 2019. Dr. Cyril Wecht, a medical examiner of true crime forensics fame, observes "the idea that people should not have to suffer. Doctors are going to take care of it. We're gonna write the prescription." The camera alternates between close-up shots of the speakers. Dr. Gupta explains, "It seems to be that we are self-medicating. We're 4.7% of the world's population. We take 80–90% of the world's oxycontin and hydrocodone." Dr. Wecht, looking a bit shocked but not surprised, shakes his head and replies "that's incredible." The camera close-up returns to Dr. Gupta as he asserts, "I'm pretty sure we don't have 80–90% of the world's pain." The audience sits in the middle of a conversation about the epidemic between two famous medical doctors. It infers that prescribing opioids drove the epidemic to its current level of crisis. The role medical doctors have in the epidemic is something that Dr. Gupta and Dr.

Wecht assert need to be reformed and reevaluated. The medical frame is affirmed here, but in a different way than it is in *Heroin(e)*. The medical field is framed as both helpful and culpable in the epidemic. This delivers even more information about the epidemic to the audience. The underlying causes include the medical profession. The scene between Dr. Wecht and Dr. Gupta offers a quick summary of how the nation got to this point and the opioid epidemic picked up speed.

TATTERED SOCIAL FABRIC AND DASHED EXPECTATIONS

In an interview with *Salon* correspondent Alli Joseph, Dr. Sanjay Gupta summarizes the additional underlying causes of the opioid epidemic and deaths of despair:

> Dashed expectations, broken dreams, unrealistic expectations, whatever it might be, seems to cause this relentless stress that is almost existential in nature. It's not just about, "I got a meeting today, I'm busy. I've got to do a presentation." It is about who you are, your identity, your value, who you represent to your parents, and your grandparents and everything. So, it's the notion of dashed expectations being really toxic, that was one of the factors that we really zeroed in on.[31]

The opioid epidemic did not arise out of nowhere. The documentaries were made around the time of a peak in the epidemic. The rise of fentanyl. Deaths from opioid overdoses in the United States at an all-time high. Digging into underlying causes and ways to stop the epidemic were certainly of interest. Getting the general public to understand the epidemic, a massive undertaking, was a palpable goal of these documentaries. Tattered social fabric is evident in both. Dashed expectations are definitely witnessed by the audience was well through the narrative arcs featured.

Anne Case, Ph.D. and Sir Angus Deaton, Ph.D., whose economic studies lead to their coining the term *deaths of despair*, are featured prominently in *One Nation Under Stress*. In their 2017 report titled *Mortality and Morbidity in the 21st Century*, Case and Deaton summarize the historical relevance and unprecedented nature of the epidemic:

> After the late 1930s, mortality fell year by year, with the exception of a pause around 1960 (which likely was attributable to the rapid increase in the prevalence of smoking in the 1930s and 1940s), with rapid decline resuming in 1970, when treatments for heart disease began to improve. In this historical context of

> almost continuous improvement, the rise in mortality in midlife is an extraordinary and unanticipated event.[32]

One Nation Under Stress uses interviews with Case and Deaton to establish the parameters for how *deaths of despair* began to garner attention in academic and governmental circles. Now they are trying to get the attention of the general public and put this heady information into an easily relatable medium. Immediately after the introduction to Angela Glass, Dr. Gupta visits Case and Deaton at Princeton University. During his initial interview with Case and Deaton, Dr. Gupta inquires about the underlying causes the pair were seeing in their research. Dashed expectations are part of the equation.

> Case: Whites are reporting poorer and poorer health. More and more pain. More and more social isolation. More depression. Along with an increase in mortality from drugs, alcohol, and suicide. There's just more morbidity, pain, social isolation.
>
> Gupta: These are the children of the people who won the world war. They were supposed to inherit the Earth.
>
> Deaton: They were promised the Earth. But they did not inherit it.
>
> Case: In every state but two, cirrhosis and alcoholic-liver disease went up. In every state, drug poisonings went up. Every state, between 1999 and 2015, suicide rates went up for people aged 25–64. If you treat people in a really shabby way for long enough, bad things happen to them. That happened to African Americans forever. And it started to happen to Whites with a high school degree or less, starting in the mid-70s, and now bad things are happening to both those groups.

Working-class Whites with a high school degree or less are a large portion of the population in places like Huntington-Cabell County in *Heroin(e)* and the stops Dr. Gupta makes in *One Nation Under Stress.* Both of the synecdochal conversion narratives featured in the documentaries fall into these demographics. According to the *National Institute on Drug Abuse,* "In 2017, West Virginia providers wrote 81.3 opioid prescriptions for every 100 persons, compared to the average U.S. rate of 58.7 prescriptions."[33] West Virginia provides a clear synecdoche for Case and Deaton's findings.

Heroin(e) and *One Nation Under Stress* cover the underlying causes and approaches to the opioid epidemic in moving ways. By literally moving alongside professional experts on the frontlines of the epidemic, they are shown a compassionate and compelling view. Lessons learned from the documentaries are many. How the epidemic got so bad is not the primary focus. Individuals who can help and were saved are featured to illustrate the complex issue of the opioid epidemic in a way that someone with no knowledge of the epidemic can grasp and adopt easily. Emotional evidence fills the time one would spend viewing the documentaries. Ultimately, the vision for finding a way out of the epidemic is to adopt the medical frame and exact compassion, not uncaring judgment or a criminality approach.

NOTES

1. "Data Overview: Overview of the Drug Overdose Epidemic: Behind the Numbers," *Opioid Overdose, Centers for Disease Control and Prevention,* 2019, https://www.cdc.gov/drugoverdose/data/index.html.

2. Jeffrey Fleishman, "Documentary Films Explore the Despair of America's Heroin and Opioid Epidemic," *The Los Angeles Times*, July 6, 2018, https://www.latimes.com/entertainment/movies/la-ca-opioids-documentaries-20180706-story.html.

3. Anne Case and Angus Deaton, "Mortality and Morbidity in the 21st Century," *Brookings Papers on Economic Activity*, Spring (2017): 398.

4. Theodore L. Caputi, "Commentary on Furr-Holden Et Al.: Drugs, Class, and Race—recent Developments in the Opioid Epidemic Call for Urgent next Steps," *Addiction* (Abingdon, England) 116, no. 3 (2021): 684.

5. Ibid, 684.

6. Ibid, 684.

7. Emma Frances Bloomfield and Angeline Sangalang, "Juxtaposition as Visual Argument: Health Rhetoric in Super Size Me and Fat Head," *Argumentation & Advocacy* 50 (3), (2014): 141.

8. "Overdose Death Rates," *National Institute on Drug Abuse, January 2019,* https://www.drugabuse.gov/related-topics/trends-statistics/overdose-death-rates.

9. Ibid.

10. "The Opioid Crisis," *Ending America's Opioid Crisis, Whitehouse.gov,* accessed January 2020, https://www.whitehouse.gov/opioids/.

11. Thomas Benson, "The Rhetorical Structure of Frederick Wiseman's Primate," *The Quarterly Journal of Speech* 71 (2), (1985): 215.

12. Ibid, 209.

13. Thomas Rosteck and Thomas S. Frentz, "The Conversion of Lila Lipscomb in Fahrenheit 9/11." In *Michael Moore and the Rhetoric of Documentary*, edited by Thomas W. Benson and Brian J. Snee (Illinois: Southern Illinois University Press, 2015), 181.

14. Bill Nichols, *Introduction to Documentary* (Bloomington: Indiana University Press, 2010), 88.

15. Bradford Vivian, "Witnessing Time: Rhetorical Form, Public Culture, and Popular Historical Education," *Rhetoric Society Quarterly* 44 (3), (2014): 213.

16. Carl R. Plantinga, *Moving Viewers American Film and the Spectator's Experience* (Berkeley: University of California Press, 2009), 6.

17. Bill Nichols, "History, Myth, and Narrative in Documentary," *Film Quarterly* 41 (1), (1987): 16.

18. Barbie Zelizer, "Finding Aids to the Past: Bearing Personal Witness to Traumatic Public Events," *Media, Culture & Society* 24 (5), (2002): 698.

19. Ibid.

20. Thomas Rosteck and Thomas S. Frentz, "The Conversion of Lila Lipscomb in Fahrenheit 9/11." In *Michael Moore and the Rhetoric of Documentary*, edited by Thomas W. Benson and Brian J. Snee (Illinois: Southern Illinois University Press, 2015), 182–83.

21. Kenneth Burke, *A Grammar of Motives* (Berkeley: University of California Press, 1945), 507–8.

22. Nicholas Kristof and Sheryl WuDunn, "Who Killed the Knapp Family?" *The New York Times,* January 9, 2020, https://nyti.ms/37Qan0A.

23. Thomas Rosteck and Thomas S. Frentz, "The Conversion of Lila Lipscomb in Fahrenheit 9/11." In *Michael Moore and the Rhetoric of Documentary*, edited by Thomas W. Benson and Brian J. Snee (Illinois: Southern Illinois University Press, 2015), 200–201.

24. "Heroin(e)," *Netflix Media Center,* 2017, https://media.netflix.com/en/only-on-netflix/80192445.

25. *One Nation Under Stress: Deaths of Despair in the United States*, directed by Marc Levin and Daphne Pinkerson (New York City, NY: HBO Documentary Films, 2019), Streaming.

26. "Understanding the Epidemic," *Opioid Overdose, Centers for Disease Control and Prevention,* 2019, https://www.cdc.gov/drugoverdose/epidemic/index.html.

27. *Heroin(e)*, directed by Elaine McMillion Sheldon (Los Angeles, CA: Netflix, 2017), Streaming.

28. Ibid.

29. National Institute on Drug Abuse, "Opioid Overdose Crisis," March 2021, https://www.drugabuse.gov/drug-topics/opioids/opioid-overdose-crisis.

30. Carl R. Plantinga, *Rhetoric and Representation in Nonfiction Film* (Cambridge, UK: Cambridge University Press, 1997), 51.

31. Alli Joseph, "Dr. Sanjay Gupta on How Income Inequality is Making Us Stressed Out," *Salon*, March 24, 2019, https://www.salon.com/2019/03/24/dr-sanjay-gupta-on-how-income-inequality-is-making-us-stressed-out/.

32. Anne Case and Angus Deaton, "Mortality and Morbidity in the 21st Century," *Brookings Papers on Economic Activity*, Spring (2017): 403.

33. "West Virginia Opioid Summary," *National Institute on Drug Abuse,* March 2019, https://www.drugabuse.gov/opioid-summaries-by-state/west-virginia-opioid-summary.

Chapter 3

Ben is Back

Mothers of the Epidemic

The winter of 2018 brought about a popular film to address the opioid epidemic. Scott Tobias of *NPR* states, "A great high-profile opioid drama is long overdue, given the enormity of the problem . . . *Ben is Back* is a useful roadmap through one of the drug-ravaged sites currently pockmarking the country."[1] While there are many films that address addiction, this is one of the only films that tackles the opioid epidemic specifically. It also has a cast and director that are common household names. It was slow at the box office, only 12.6 million according to *IMDB,* but it is still the most noteworthy due to its casting and the particular focus upon the opioid epidemic. Oddly, Julia Roberts's performance was not given any major awards, in spite of her receiving rave reviews from A.O. Scott of *The New York Times* and high user ratings, 82 percent, on *Rotten Tomatoes.* Perhaps this is telling of our nation's slow response to stymie the tide of the epidemic and affix our collective focus upon ending the complex underlying causes.

With a stellar cast, writer and director Peter Hedges's *Ben is Back* deliver on what Tobias remarked was overdue. Moving performances and details revealing information about the epidemic along the way win it critical praise for the film's realism. The realism addresses what A.O. Scott of *The New York Times* describes as a challenge for the film. Scott explains, "one of the cruelties of addiction is the way it strips away individuality, making all addicts' stories the same." The film brings the audience into the epidemic with a powerful synecdoche drama. Through the point of view of Holly, played by Julia Roberts, the mother of an addict, Hedges' film informs and persuades with the story of a family on Christmas Eve. Scott's review states, "part of her [Holly] terror—and ours, on her behalf—comes from the sense that she is radically and brutally alone, and that the hundreds of thousands of parents in her situation are too."[2] Ironically, as I will explore in the analysis of the film,

Ben is Back demonstrates that individuals impacted by this epidemic are not alone and serves as a synecdoche for the broader social crisis.

The family of Ben Burns, a young addict who returns home from rehab for Christmas, lends to the authenticity the film is praised for. Ben is played by Hedges's son in real life, Lucas Hedges. Courtney B. Vance is Ben's stepfather. Kathryn Newton plays Ben's sister. Julia Roberts's performance is powerful. The dynamic between Roberts and the other actors carries a backstory that does not need to be said aloud, it taps into the audiences' preconceived notions and knowledge of the epidemic well. Stigma about drug use is addressed head on throughout the film and the synecdoche of one mother's compassion and unending love argues that we ought to extend the same in real life while approaching the opioid epidemic. The script is thoughtful and purposefully unveils issues and information about the epidemic with each plot turn. More specifically, Ben's mother, Holly, lends a rhetorical lift as being the main point of identification for the audience. *Ben is Back* functions rhetorically in important ways in this popular representation of the opioid epidemic. In this chapter, I analyze how the discourses of the opioid epidemic manifest in a popular film. I explore the synecdoche of the broader epidemic the film presents, themes in the film, and detail the cultural significance of the turns the narrative takes. The film acts like a mirror, reflecting back the epidemic which our society has yet to find a way out of. No cure is in sight. And we will not save everyone from its deadly grip.

As a rhetorical text, it is important to note what is selected as important information about the epidemic and *how* the film reflects the epidemic back to us. My goal in this chapter is to interrogate *Ben is Back* as a narrative that simultaneously informs and reflects back to the audience the state of the opioid epidemic when the film debuted in 2018. The film acts as a rhetorical site of production and reflection, working in a bivalent fashion from the facts of the epidemic to the fictional account that is the subject of the film. *Ben is Back* visualizes and narrativizes what the epidemic *is,* how to *view* the epidemic, and how we ought to *feel* it. The rhetorical articulation of what the epidemic *is*, as well as whom the audience is invited to most strongly engage with, the character of Holly, makes the film a significant text in its own right.

RHETORIC OF FILM

Understanding the discursive contours of the opioid epidemic requires the inclusion popular media representations. Lara Stache states, "Media give us complex and persuasive messages about the work in which we live and allow us to make sense of the world around us."[3] There have been numerous documentaries that tackle the subject of the opioid epidemic. A few of them are analyzed in other chapters of this book. Many are of critical acclaim, such as *Heroin(e).* Jeffrey Fleishman of the *Los Angeles Times* reported in July of 2018 about the "surge in documentaries in recent years" that zoom in on "drug marketing, prescribing doctors, border patrol agents, drug rehab centers, wrecked families, traffickers, and soaring addiction rates in small towns from Vermont to Kentucky."[4] A Hollywood, fictional account of a family in the throes of the opioid epidemic allows for an unencumbered, slightly cathartic, and much safer space to process the epidemic.

Popular films are productive sites in which traumatic topics and anxieties the Nation is experiencing as a whole may be engaged. The medium of film affords a narrative that assists with understanding and working through trauma. Claire Sisco King writes, "narratives about traumatic experience can be understood as rhetorical efforts to rescript the past, if not to change its outcomes, then to change it meanings."[5] Furthermore, films are sites where an audience can grapple with cultural anxieties and trauma from a safer distance.[6] The opioid epidemic has had deadly consequences. Carl R. Plantinga finds film "can enlarge understanding and sympathy for characters whose lives and experiences extend far beyond our own experience, and thus enhance our sentimental education. It is not the spectator's attitude toward particular persons or events that are at issue here, but the general training of perception and judgment," which articulates the epidemic in a relatable way.[7] With the whole country reeling, the epidemic is much easier to comprehend as a synecdoche through an approachable medium with an A-list celebrity front and center. Just with the casting of Julia Roberts as the central character, *Ben is Back* secures a large audience to be informed and persuaded about a particular way to view the opioid epidemic and addiction writ large. The film is messy and complicated, but the message it is able to deliver through the main character is simple: love equals hope for this epidemic.

Synecdoche, in the Burkean sense, is a related representation of the material condition. Synecdoche is a part representing a whole. *Ben is Back* stands in as an approachable toe-hold into a complex epidemic by way of a compelling narrative and family drama makes it highly relatable.[8] The film, which represents part of the epidemic, stands in for the whole for the viewer's experience. The narrative is centered upon a mother trying desperately to save her son from his opioid addiction. The mother is a sympathetic character who is safe to identify with. She is white, middle class, and adores her four children. Her son—Ben—is white, clean cut, and looks like a good kid. Ben is also shown early in the film being adored by his younger half-siblings and goofing around with them. The family looks to be functioning well with Ben after he returns to his middle-class life after rehab for Christmas. But, dig a little deeper, and the plot reveals that Ben and his mother were once living in poverty, they were abandoned by his biological father when he was young, and it was an injury and careless physician who started his drug addiction through prescription opioids. The way Ben's addiction begins also makes the film much more relatable and safer to connect with.

This family drama style of subtle nods to a troubled past is typical of the director. Though only one family's experience of the epidemic is the focus, the story of this particular family can stand in and represent the experience of the whole of the epidemic an engaging way. Director Peter Hedges is well known for capturing family drama in moving and compelling ways. The film also gets the audience to wonder what they would do or compare the ways in which their lives have been impacted by the epidemic. The rhetorical dynamics of the film emotionally engage the audience in meaningful ways. Stache's study of the series *Breaking Bad,* a popular series reflecting upon another rampant drug issue plaguing the country right alongside this one, closes with the sentiment that we need quality media that "requires us to think about the way our world works outside of the fictional universe."[9] *Ben is Back* invites the audience to think about the world outside of the film as well and question how far you would go to save a loved one from addiction.

The film orders the importance of particular facets of the massive epidemic. According to John A. Bateman and Karl-Heinrich Schmidt, "Films appear to more or less directly inform viewers which pieces of information have to be brought together, which not, and when."[10] The microcosm, or synecdochal representation, put forward in the narrative selects particular focal points from the larger whole, frames the information through the point of view of a particular character who is safely relatable, and buffers the emotional impact of the human side of the epidemic. Films articulate those pieces into an emotional topography to guide the viewer through the plot. Plantinga explains, "Emotions provide narrative information that is necessary for audiences to follow the narrative. In extra-filmic life, our emotions focus our attention on salient details of the environment; the emotions elicited in a film function similarly, often drawing our attention to those elements that the film constructs as essential to understanding the narrative."[11] The topography of emotion is explored in the following pages along with an interrogation of the film's cues that shape the experience of the opioid epidemic the audience is invited to.

The audience is strongly invited to identify the opioid epidemic by identifying with a mother's love for her child. How she is doing whatever she can to save her son, the film is framing the epidemic as a medical plight—pitting a mother against a disease for which there may be no cure—and thereby getting the audience to identify with the love in the situation. Identification, in a rhetorical sense of the word, is about *belonging* and *consubstantiality.*[12] The film finds ways to bring the audience in and find the character they like or are more like. They then are invited to identify with the epidemic on the level of that particular character. The characters having a complex backstory that involves dynamics of race, class, and gender, make the choices available for the audience dynamic enough to allow identification for a large swath of the audience. *Ben is Back* tells the story of a middle-class family on Christmas Eve in suburban America during the opioid epidemic. There is a deeper story of pain that the mother and son are experiencing that fuels the addiction and sets a dark pall on the hope of Christmas and family togetherness that Rockwellian-narrative would have us believing is there at the beginning of the film.

VISUALIZING THE EPIDEMIC THROUGH COMPELLING NARRATIVE

The vocabulary of the camera does a lot of rhetorical work to show what the epidemic is and who it impacts. Anyone involved in the life of a sufferer suffers along with their afflicted loved one. The film opens on a Rockwellian scene. Almost like vintage Christmas time postcards, the first few scenes look picturesque. Snow is on the ground and the opening scene is pastoral, harkening back to a simpler time of farms and quaint small towns. The wide shots in the opening sequence feature a snow covered, rustic, East coast looking barn in the center of the screen. The scene then cuts to a quaint cemetery. Next, the main street in a small town is shown. Then a quick cut to a small pharmacy that cuts fairly quickly to the exterior of a church. Though picturesque, something feels off about these early scenes that feel like old-time Christmas postcards. The scene cuts to a close-up of the first character the audience sees: Holly Burns. The camera zooms out from her face, setting up that this is the character's point of view the audience will follow throughout the duration of the film, and then cuts to her point of view to a choir singing Christmas hymns.

The experiences Holly has with the epidemic guides the audience through the basics of the opioid epidemic. Just as the pastoral East coast town establishes, the early scenes of Holly in church demonstrate a happy family that is about to face a major challenge. This is a subtle reference to the areas of the country that were the hardest hit. The epidemic was initially worst in the southwest and eastern parts of the United States. Holly is watching her daughter Ivy sing for the Christmas eve performance. Her younger two children are eager to leave church and get home after a long practice. The camera shifts to a handheld and cuts to a hooded figure walking up to a home. The change in camera demonstrates a few things. It ushers in the destabilization factor into the film. The figure in the snow will destabilize this Rockwellian scene the first few scenes have established. The harsh sound of the snow crunching under his boots is a stark contrast from the Christmas carols and jovial children in the church. The oscillation between the steady cam that is focused on Holly and the handheld that focuses on the hooded figure lurking around the family home windows foreshadows the destabilization and chaos that is about to strike. The handheld camera represents the stabilization that the character lurking around the family home presents to the scene.

Sounds and visuals reinforce the identification with Holly. The opening visuals and sounds of Holly are joyful, picturesque, and represent American ideals. The scene then cuts back to Holly and her children driving in the family Subaru. They are funny, joking around with one another, and seem tightknit. This is contrast to the switch back to the handheld camera aesthetic as the scene returns to the hooded figure trying to enter a home with no success. The family dog is barking from inside the house. This shift from steady cam to handheld ruptures the Rockwellian scenes the film opens on. Upon Holly and her children pulling up to their house, the audience finally gets a look at the hooded figure's face. Here the audience is introduced formally to Ben who has returned home from rehab for Christmas. Holly's point of view is reinforced through a gasp. It escapes her unwittingly as she slams the brakes at the sight of the hooded figure. The joy in the family car is cut off abruptly. It shifts to a tense and peculiar blend of excitement and nerves as the audience watches through the windshield of the Subaru a reunion between mother and son.

IDENTIFYING (WITH) THE OPIOID EPIDEMIC

Information about the epidemic itself is interspersed throughout the plot. Identifying what the epidemic *is* presents itself as the plot unfolds. The medical frame is introduced right away and is part of developing Holly's character as a compassionate, yet fierce, advocate for her son's health and recovery. Early on in the film, shortly after Ben returns home, Holly takes him to the mall to go shopping for clothes to attend church for Christmas Eve mass. Ben had shown up with no bag, which should have been a sign that he left rehab without permission or against recommendation, but Holly is too overjoyed at seeing her son healthy and sober to notice. Holly approaches an elderly man in the food court. She asks if the man remembers Ben who is sitting a few tables away from them. The old man shakes his head and is clearly in the later stages of dementia. Throughout their short interaction, the story of how Ben gets addicted to pain pills at fourteen after a minor snowboarding injury unfolds. Holly was told by the doctor that the pills were safe, important for Ben's recovery from the injury, and not addictive. The doctor kept on increasing Ben's dose. Holly concludes the conversation by saying, "You can pretend like you don't remember. But I won't forget. I hope you die a horrible death." The sweet and caring mother, Holly, becomes overwhelmed by her anger at the doctor who robbed her son of a normal life because of careless prescribing practices. This is key to the medical frame of the opioid epidemic as well as the level of compassion that is necessary for turning the tide of the epidemic. Holly is committed not only because she is a devoted mother, but because she recognizes the cause of Ben's addiction was not through his choices or actions, but due to being lied to about a medically prescribed substance that is actually highly addictive.

In spite of Holly's compassion and the medical frame, showing the potency of the addiction and dependency to opioids is also necessary to properly inform the audience of the hold that these drugs have on sufferers. The level of scrutiny and the ways a mother has to be vigilant around her son is demonstrated in a few powerful scenes. After leaving a Narcotics Anonymous meeting to reward Ben for sharing candidly in the meeting, Holly takes him to a clothing store to shop for clothes for the Christmas Eve service. Holly checks his pockets before letting him go in the changing room. At the beginning of the film there is an agreement that Ben can stay with his family for twenty-four hours, if he has a clean urine analysis, and then he must return to complete his rehab. Holly grabs Ben and tells him, "For the next twenty-four hours, you are mine. All mine. Got it." Checking Ben's pockets, even after she has been around him nonstop, demonstrates the level of vigilance and distrust in the relationship. Holly starts to panic after the door closes because Ben says the joke, "You didn't check my shoes," right after the changing door closes. Holly is slamming on the door and yelling for him to open it. Ben finally opens the door and slips a small bag of drugs into her hand. Holly is hitting his chest and yelling when a store clerk asks them to leave the store during their fight. Most of the scenes are focused on Holly's interactions with Ben to reinforce the audience's identification with her as the main character as well as her perspective of the epidemic.

Identification and ensuring the synecdoche sticks with the audience is largely crafted through Julia Roberts performance as Holly. Plantinga explains how a well-known and well-loved actress can do extra work for the film by crafting allegiance with particular characters, "*Allegiance* with characters is another essential component of the structure of engagement. Allegiance has a stronger moral and affective component than alignment, and is less a structure of the text than a response of spectators to characters. Allegiance results from the spectator's moral evaluation of characters."[13] Furthermore, Holly being played by Julia Roberts does particular work to drive that allegiance and moral valuation of the situations in the film even more. Plantinga remarks "The 'star system,' casting a big name in a role, can partially account for audience allegiances to particular characters as well."[14] A few private moments of Holly in front of mirrors or close-ups of her reacting to Ben's remarks show her inner terror and turmoil, which ultimately reinforce the audience's identification with Holly, and progress the general feelings of frustration with the epidemic. Through this strong identification, the audience can more easily adopt Holly's approach to the epidemic and those suffering from opioid use disorders. Particularly after the scene where you see this mild mannered mother of four enraged and saying terrible things to her son's former physician, blame is placed squarely upon the careless practices of doctors prescribing these deadly and highly addictive substances.

The stakes of the epidemic are put clearly with the following scene. The rupture that Ben's coming home before completing rehab manifests in another scene. The picturesque image of a snow-covered cemetery from the opening sequence of the film is revisited with Holly. She drives over to the cemetery, drags Ben out of the car, and calmly asks, "So where? Where do you want to be?" Ben is uncomfortable and looking like he does not want to be there. "Just tell me son, where you want me to bury you? I'll wait all day." Ben says, "I'm not going to die." Holly, "At this rate you will. And soon." Holly doesn't cry. She is angry. Furious in fact. Like so many families in the United States, the cycle of drug use, overdose, and rehab are not new for Holly's family. The audience gets the sense that she has done this too many times before to cry. Ben is calm too. He seems sympathetic to his mother, but not remorseful for his drug use. Even though the film is sharing a stark reality of the epidemic, mothers burying their sons, it is still presented through the compassionate lens of Holly's perspective. She is still fighting and will continue until her son is dead. Holly's compassion is never-ending for her son. A fitting synecdoche for this type of epidemic.

Socioeconomics as a major factor of the epidemic comes into the plot about halfway through the film. While Holly and Ben are out together at a late-night diner, it becomes clear that Ben is Holly's top priority. She has completely abandoned her other three children and husband for the sake of devoting her energy to keeping Ben clean while he is at home. After a heated phone conversation between Holly and her husband Neal concludes, Ben says of Neal, "He's a bit of a dick." Holly replies, "No, I can think or say about him whatever I want because he is my husband, and I love him, but you . . . God, you clearly don't get it. You're here, and without Neal, you wouldn't be. Mm, don't be so sure. How many rehabs is it now? I couldn't've paid for it. Insurance won't anymore. The government doesn't give a fuck. And, heaven help you if you're poor, which, because of Neal, we aren't anymore. He took out a second mortgage on the house to pay for you this time. The only thing you should say about Neal is thank you." In this brief scene, Holly summarizes the issue of socioeconomics in the opioid epidemic. Social inequity, the feelings of being abandoned by the government, forsaken by health insurance plans, and money being one of the few salvations to pay for private rehabilitation as a final glimmer of hope. The scene is a powerful one.

Overdose reversal as a way to keep a loved one alive long enough to complete rehab is part of what is included as the picture of the opioid epidemic. It also reinforces the medicalization narrative and public health framing of the broader issue. Ben is also home from rehabilitation and not jail. This also rhetorically reinforces how we as a society ought to approach the epidemic. Naloxone, an overdose reversal medication, enters the picture as a key part of the plot. Ben gives Holly the slip during their period of twenty-four hours before he is to return to finish out rehab. Holly goes to visit the mother of a girl who died recently of an overdose. Ben was the girl's dealer and got her involved with drugs. Beth gives Holly a Naloxone kit that she did not have the opportunity to use to save her own child. Holly says, "I am such a smug bitch. I never thought I'd need this. I can't do this." Beth gives instructions to Holly for how to use it and says it should still be good. Holly says, "But, if you couldn't save Maggie . . ." Beth interrupts, "We can't save them. But you'll hate yourself if you don't try." Naloxone is a medication that interrupts the effects of opioids by blocking opioid receptors in the brain. The medicine, in the version that Holly receives, is a kit that you assemble and then given through the nose as a spray. The audience receives the tutorial from a bereaved mother to another mother desperately trying to give her son as many chances as necessary to get him out of the throws of addiction.

The role that pharmacies and fraught policies play in the epidemic, many of which have been updated since the film's release, are featured next. Pharmacies and patients unwittingly following doctor's orders that lead to their demise strengthens the medicalization of the narrative and public health frame. It locates blame for the epidemic in another powerful scene featuring Holly and her anger at the system that devastated her family. Holly visits the local pharmacy to receive a newer dose of Naloxone because the one she received was close to its expiration date. The pharmacist tells Holly she cannot replace it because, "It's our policy not to encourage irresponsible behavior." That is one of the major misunderstandings about the medication Naloxone. The audience, if they had this misperception of Naloxone, would be receiving more nuanced information through the film. Holly, furious, replies to the pharmacist, "Alright, well, then why don't you discontinue the oxys, the Perc 30s, and the . . .the . . . the benzo cheerios or whatever you call them!" The interaction reveals that pharmacies all over the country are willingly filling prescriptions for opioids, feeding the flames of the epidemic, and greed of pharmaceutical companies that are easy to get hooked on. Holly makes it clear to the pharmacist, and thereby the audience, that the pharmacy and others are indeed encouraging irresponsible behavior with every opioid prescription filled. Yet, the pharmacist is not willing to replace an overdose reversal medicine that is exclusively used to save a life and is not addictive. The strong identification with Holly is key for receiving this information and identifying Naloxone as a positive in the fight against the epidemic.

A MOTHER'S LOVE TO FRAME THE EPIDEMIC

Holly's love for her son is crucial to the movement of the film and the movement of the audience to see the epidemic through her eyes. The scene with Holly and the doctor showed her fierce commitment and where the rage came from. Ben is not someone who fell into addiction as a choice or a failing of moral character. Part of Holly's never-ending compassion for Ben is due to her belief that it is not his fault. It also informs the audience that many of the people in the thralls of opioid addiction did not choose addiction. Like Ben, many were just following the orders of a medical doctor for a legitimate injury and medical need. They unwittingly, following the orders of a doctor, became addicts to a pain killer that was medically advisable for their condition. The repetition of moments like this in the film supports the medicalization narrative and public health framing of compassionate solutions to the epidemic.

During the twenty-four hours at home, Holly is treating Ben to some snacks at a convenience mart when he gives her the slip. Holly was out looking for Ben all night long and did not let on to her husband, Neal, that she had lost track of Ben. As day breaks on Christmas morning, Holly finally calls Neal, "I lost him. I didn't want to tell you. I was lying to you. I looked everywhere for him. I tried." Neal replies, "I know you did." The audience gets the sense that this is not the first time that Holly has covered for Ben to her husband Neal. Holly starts to cry as she admits to Neal, "I lost him a long time ago. And I am tired. I don't know what to do." Neal reassures her by saying, "Tell me where you are. I'm coming to get you. And we'll find him together." It is the first time in the movie that Holly actually allows herself to cry and to admit that she needs comfort. At a time when Ben's character is coming across as rather unsympathetic and difficult to connect with, all of the work that the film does to connect the audience with Holly's character is vital to continue the medical, compassionate framing of the epidemic. Neal's response reinforces the framing and demonstrates the need for family support during challenges such as this situation the family finds itself in. Many stories about the epidemic and those whom are lost to it are ones lacking this support. That lack of support is part of what drive deaths of despair and the road to addiction in the United States in general. *Ben is Back* actually features a story with hope, compassion, and familial support that too many in reality lack.

The legal frame only appears in the film twice. It does not upend the compassionate, medical frame that the audience identifies with Holly's approach to her son. This is a tidy synecdoche for the epidemic as a whole. The legal frame does enter in a minor way and is not acted upon. Ben is never in legal trouble for his addiction struggles. Holly reaches a breaking point on Christmas morning when she calls Neal. Holly finally realizes that she needs help with Ben and cannot keep him safe on her own. Ben is a danger to himself on his own. Holly arrives at the nearest police station. The officer at the front counter asks for a description, Holly slams her hands on their window and yells, "No, no, there's no time for that. Could you please just find my son and arrest him!" This is the first time that something other than letting Ben have a solely medical solution is proposed. Holly turns to the police in a moment of crisis after looking for Ben all night to no avail. It is out of desperation and the willingness to do whatever it takes to keep her son safe and alive long enough to medically recover.

The privilege of Ben's identity had come into play earlier in the film. Holly's second husband Neal, Ben's stepfather, is African American. In an early scene in the film, while Holly is imploring Neal to let Ben stay with them for Christmas, Neal states plainly, "If he were black, he would be in jail by now. We said we weren't going to do this again." Because Ben is white, he is able to avoid incarceration more easily while his mother keeps fighting for him. Holly's second marriage to Neal, Ben's stepfather, brought their income level up significantly enough so Ben has been able to avoid some of the harsher realities of addiction by accessing private rehabilitation facilities and mental health support. The legal frame is only present in the film twice to make points about the epidemic and to inform the audience about the dynamics at play with the opioid epidemic in particular.

The racial iniquities that plague American society are nodded at once again in the film. Not all drug use in America is approached the same and the film acknowledges it briefly. A scene was cut from the film in the sequence where Holly loses track of him and is looking for him. Holly approaches an African American woman sitting on a sidewalk. Holly asks her if she has seen her son and shows a picture of Ben on her phone. That portion remains in the film. The part where the woman asks Holly, "Where were you? Where were you when my baby was lost?" The director, Peter Hedges, references the crack-cocaine epidemic of the 1980s that disproportionately impacted the African American community and was largely ignored by the Government in productive ways in this scene. Instead, the film shows Holly's interaction with the woman on the sidewalk in a briefer form. Holly inquires if she has seen her son, shows her a picture of him on her mobile, and then she says what direction Ben went in. This inequity of how the various drug use issues in our country is approached is important for Hedges. Ultimately, Hedges decides to cut the scene from the film because it detracted from the journey Holly was on and would distract from the overdose that was around the corner.

Sufferers of opioid use disorder often experience being "dope sick" and the film explores that through a former friend of Ben's named Spider. Dope sicknesses is the medical condition of seeking a substance to stave off a whole host of symptoms that are painful, rather than seeking a substance for euphoric effects. Spider shows up briefly in the first third and the last third of the film. The bookending of the character drives the medicalization and public health framing further and emphasizes the importance of the never-ending well of compassion that Holly represents to defeat the epidemic. Spider and Holly connect the second time after she has lost track of Ben. Holly finds Spider in order to ask him where he thinks Ben might be so she can go look in more places. Spider represents the sufferer who did not have a support system, did not have access to rehabilitation, and is fully in the throes of addiction with no hope of recovery. His real name is not Spider, but it demonstrates for the audience the ways in which addiction can rob a person of what makes them an individual.

Spider is the foil to Ben in many ways and synecdoche to how things could go if there is no social or familial support. Ben has support and a family who keeps on funding his attempts to turn his life around and be clear from addiction. Spider has been fully enveloped and the new name marks that full transformation. Holly offers the opioids she confiscates from Ben in an earlier scene to Spider in exchange for information on how to find Ben. Spider explains to Holly that he does not want to get high, instead, he just wants to "get right" and not suffer the symptoms of being dope sick anymore. As Spider exits Holly's vehicle, she yells after him, "Go call your mother!" The perspective to take is affirmed through this line from Holly. The hope would be that, if Ben were as lost as Spider, that he would still reach out to Holly and recognize her never-ending love for him.

The framing of the epidemic through what our culture and society values, the enduring compassion and love of a mother, is hammered into the minds of the audience throughout the film. This scene also serves the objective to inform the audience of the power of opioids. It introduces the reality of chasing more opioids being about feeling well, avoiding being sick, and not just about the derogatory, negative associations that go along with the pursuit of getting high. This is firmly within the vein of the medical frame and demonstrates the physical symptoms of opioid use disorder for the audience.

Informing the audience about an overdose is vital for understanding the epidemic. The medical and compassion frames are reinforced in the overdose scenes of the film. What an overdose can look like is featured in two scenes of the film. Both are responded to with more chances to turn over a new leaf, are presented with medical options, and the undying compassion of a mother's love toward her son. The first overdose scene is brief and not visually demonstrated. Ben's first overdose is discussed during the Narcotics Anonymous meeting early on in the film. While it is not shown to the audience, it is, however, foreshadowed early into Ben's brief time visiting his family. The scene discussed in the Narcotics Anonymous meeting is foreshadowed in an earlier time in the film shortly after Holly makes a deal with her husband Neal that allows Ben to stay with them for Christmas and then return promptly to rehab. Holly had been distracted by her other children, becomes concerned, and peers through a partially open door into Ben's bedroom to check on him. Holly discovers Ben lying on the ground. She immediately has a panicked look on her face as she throws the bedroom door open, only to find, much to her relief, that Ben was not actually unconscious. Ben's face changes from the joy of playing with the family dog, Ponce, to a look of offense at his mother's response. Ponce is referenced in the story told during his share in the meeting. Ben's relationship and closeness with Ponce becomes clearer through the share as he recounts that he is only alive because of the love of his family, particularly their dog. Ponce was the hero who kept licking him and pawing him to keep him awake enough to get help. Holly found him, got him to the emergency room in time to be resuscitated, and Ponce is the big reason why Ben is on day 77 of his sobriety during the share at the Narcotics Anonymous meeting. It is moving to have the scene alluded to rather than shown. It is part of their story that leads to Holly's hypervigilance during Ben's stay. It shows the side of Ben before sobriety and the beauty, humor, and brightness of a son who is the person Holly keeps fighting tirelessly for.

The next, more developed overdose scene, occurs at the conclusion of the film. It is a highly emotional scene. It also seems to be the inevitable conclusion of the film after seeing Ben devolve under Holly's supervision. The barn from the opening scene, old-time Christmas postcard sequence is revisited. This is the site where Ben overdoses after giving Holly the slip during their time together, where Ben is supposed to be under constant surveillance, but plays on her emotions by acting like he is being a good, complimentary son. Ben goes to the same pharmacy where Holly was denied a Naloxone exchange to retrieve a clean needle to shoot up heroin. Commentary on the hypocrisy of the pharmacist is highlighted in this brief scene. The irony of the pharmacy visit is not lost on the viewer. Ben receives the syringe with no resistance. The policies that denied Holly access to a Naloxone replacement that would "encourage irresponsible behavior" are the same ones that allow an addict access to a syringe to overdose with.

The synecdoche reaches its climax at the end of the film. The stakes and hope of the epidemic are demonstrated in a dramatic fashion that fully test Holly's resolve. Ben then continues his journey to the barn. The disruption of the Rockwellian scene takes its final and most heavy twist. Ben leaves

Ponce, the family dog, in Holly's car with a note that says to contact Holly to get the dog home. The scene cuts to Holly at the police station where she receives a phone call from an older man who found the car, note, and Ponce locked inside. Holly shows up to the home of the man who phoned her after finding Ponce in the car with the note. Dramatic piano music is in the foreground. The piano fades as Holly lets Ponce out of the car. Ponce barks and races to the barn. The lack of music marks an emotional shift in the scene. Holly follows Ponce to find an unresponsive, supine, and vaguely blue looking Ben. Holly cries as she starts to shake Ben, "Honey! Wake up, Ben. Wake up, Ben! Honey." As Holly wipes away her tears, her demeanor changes as she removes a Naloxone kit from her pocket. Holly takes a breath and says, "Okay, we've got this. Come on, hang in there. Come on, come back to me. Wake up! Wake up!" Holly removes the tourniquet from his arm and begins rescue breathing. Ponce is barking and pacing just outside of the shot. The shot is a close-up of Holly's actions as she attempts to reverse Ben's overdose. Holly stops the rescue breathing and lays her head on his chest. Ben finally inhales and starts to open his eyes. It is a fairly tight close-up shot that frames Holly's face over Ben's. As he starts to return, Holly's face is a torrid mix of relief, despair, frustration, and love. Holly's compassion is never-ending, which sends the message that this type of compassion is what it will take to combat the opioid epidemic.

SYNECDOCHE FOR A SOCIAL CRISIS

Ben is Back provides an optimistic view of the opioid epidemic for the audience. The film is optimistic in a few key ways and the character of Holly is central to all of them. Holly provides a continual well of hope, love, and she will stop at nothing to keep her son alive. Unlike the character Spider, Ben has Holly. Holly is always supportive, loving, and there for Ben. Ben's socioeconomic status also provides expensive rehabilitation facility access that not all those who suffer would be able to utilize. Holly also manages to rescue Ben from death twice: once with a quick response to keep him awake and get him to the emergency room and the second instance with the use of overdose-reversing medication. The key to Ben's survival is his support system. That lesson is not off from what the facts about the opioid epidemic are.

Holly is a synecdoche that the director, Peter Hedges, hopes the audience will adopt as their stance on the opioid epidemic and those suffering. The suffering includes those personally experiencing the impact of addiction themselves through using opioids and those who love them. Shortly after the film's release in a *Los Angeles Times* article, Hedges himself speaks about the film and his purpose behind it, "So, yes, I wrote a script called 'Ben Is

Back' that I got to make with a bunch of remarkable artists and craftspeople. It's an urgent attempt to deal with the heroin/opioid epidemic that is ravaging our country."[15] It is also a moving medicalized narrative about too much love, which Hedges remarks is his "favorite kind of love," and is the kind of love required to overcome the opioid epidemic.

Holly loves her son so much that she gives him chance after chance. The film justifies this response, not only through the mother-son dynamic, but through the medical frame. Repeatedly, Ben is treated by Holly like a patient. Someone requiring medical care, attention, and unending love to ensure his survival. If Ben is alive, then Holly has another chance to get him fully recovered. The focus on Holly allows for a more comfortable character to identify with. A mother's love is also a familiar trope that the audience can comprehend amidst picking up additional information about the complex opioid epidemic. Seeing the epidemic through the lens of a mother's love affirms the medical frame and leaves little doubt for a compassionate approach to those afflicted with opioid use disorder.

NOTES

1. Scott Tobias, "*Ben is Back:* Well-Acted Addiction Drama Loses Its Way," *NPR,* December 6, 2018, https://www.npr.org/2018/12/06/673324119/ben-is-back-well-acted-addiction-drama-loses-its-way.
2. A. O. Scott, "*Ben is Back* Review: A Mother and Son Face the Horrors of Addiction," *The New York Times,* December 5, 2018, https://www.nytimes.com/2018/12/05/movies/ben-is-back-review.html.
3. Lara C. Stache, *Breaking Bad: A Cultural History* (Lanham: Rowman & Littlefield, 2017), xvi.
4. Jeffrey Fleishman, "Documentary Films Explore the Despair of America's Heroin and Opioid Epidemic," *Los Angeles Times,* July 6, 2018, https://www.latimes.com/entertainment/movies/la-ca-opioids-documentaries-20180706-story.html.
5. Claire Sisco King, "Rogue Waves, Remakes, and Resurrections: Allegorical Displacement and Screen Memory in *Poseidon,*" *Quarterly Journal of Speech*, 94 (4), (2008): 431.
6. Kendall R. Phillips, *Dark Directions: Romero, Craven, Carpenter, and the Modern Horror Film* (Carbondale: Southern Illinois University Press, 2012), 2.
7. Carl R. Plantinga, *Moving Viewers American Film and the Spectator's Experience* (Berkeley: University of California Press, 2009), 203.
8. Kenneth Burke, "Four Master Tropes." In *A Grammar of Motives* (Berkeley: University of California Press, 1945), 506.
9. Lara C. Stache, *Breaking Bad: A Cultural History* (Lanham: Rowman & Littlefield, 2017), 151.

10. John A. Bateman and Karl-Heinrich Schmidt, *Multimodal Film Analysis How Films Mean* (New York: Routledge, 2012), 1.

11. Carl R. Plantinga, *Moving Viewers American Film and the Spectator's Experience* (Berkeley: University of California Press, 2009), 6.

12. Kenneth Burke, *A Rhetoric of Motives* (Berkeley: University of California Press, 1969), 21.

13. Carl R. Plantinga, *Moving Viewers American Film and the Spectator's Experience* (Berkeley: University of California Press, 2009), 107.

14. Ibid, 108.

15. Peter Hedges, "'Ben Is Back' Writer-Director Peter Hedges Uncovers the Heroic Core of Broken Women," *Los Angeles Times,* December 18, 2018, https://www.latimes.com/entertainment/envelope/la-en-mn-writing-ben-is-back-20181203-story.html.

Chapter 4

Defining Trump's America through Crisis

Remarks on Combating the Opioid Crisis

It was time to make America great again. By any means necessary. Even if it meant using the death penalty more. The speech titled *Remarks on Combating the Opioid Crisis* was delivered on March 19, 2018, and came shortly after the President declared the opioid epidemic a public health emergency in October 2017.[1] It may seem ironic to use death to defeat the deadly opioid epidemic, but that is one—of the more alarming—points in Trump's plan to defeat the opioid epidemic. First Lady Melania even made the opioid crisis one of her signature issues. The White House seemed committed to ending the crisis and Trump swore it would be gone shortly after he took office. The opioid epidemic challenged Trump's predecessors and was not going to be vanquished by the forty-fifth president either.

The year 2017, the deadliest thus far in the epidemic, demanded even more be done at the highest levels of government. Trump was the first president to declare the opioid epidemic a public health emergency and signed the largest funding bill in history, with bipartisan support, toward ending "drug scourge."[2] In the speech, Trump discusses the impacts the opioid epidemic has had on families and the pressures it has put on law enforcement. He highlights parts of his plan, which include: drug education campaigns for children, funding access for local governments to purchase overdose-reversing medication, incentives for drug companies to create nonaddictive pain medications, increasing penalties for drug dealers and doctors up to the death penalty, and more. It also set up an opportunity for Trump to rally his base and further talks of his reelection. He even goes so far as to say, "I don't want to leave at the end of seven years and have this problem, okay? . . . A lot of voters in this room. I see that. Thank you. No, we're going to solve this problem."[3] The setting of the speech is in New Hampshire, where Trump's campaigning for office began, and is also a state that has been particularly impacted by the opioid epidemic. New Hampshire had the "third highest drug overdose in the nation in 2016."[4] The president had been touting harsher punishments for drug offenses the year leading up to this speech and the details of his plan to end the epidemic.[5] This portion of the speech is the most prominent and most problematic. The user of the opioid is portrayed as a victim in the speech to the menacing foes that Trump cites as responsible for killing so many Americans.

Trump's administration made "ending America's opioid crisis" a priority roughly one year after he took office. The White House's official web page devoted to the subject touts, "Since President Donald J. Trump issued a nationwide call to action, the results offer hope that we can solve the worst drug crisis in U.S. history."[6] On the official Whitehouse website page titled *Ending America's Opioid Crisis*, Trump's administration purports their nationwide call to action yields results that "offer hope that we can solve the worst drug crisis in U.S. history."[7] The speech marked the official plans and policies to end the opioid crisis. But it also, just as importantly, provides a clear view into how President Trump views the crisis, the nation, and his solutions are telling for where he ultimately places praise and blame.

On its face, President Trump's speech about combating the opioid crisis could appear to be about policy. It is not a deliberative speech about seeking policy approval, but rather an epideictic speech, extolling the morals and values of President Trump's vision of the United States. Trump moves through the speech offering praise and blame for the opioid epidemic. While policy and the President's plan to end the crisis are important features of the speech, looking more deeply with a close textual analysis, the speech yields more of an epideictic sentiment. The speech also proves to be a tenuous rhetorical treatment of the opioid epidemic. One divided between approaching the epidemic as a security threat and a major public health crisis. I will demonstrate how Trump defines his vision of America through the lens of a crisis. Furthermore, by leveraging the moment of a crisis, President Trump offers further evidence and support for his campaign promises and policy stances that are loosely related to the opioid crisis.

PRESIDENTIAL EPIDEICTIC RHETORIC GETS TOUGH ON DRUGS

Epideictic rhetoric is defined as a genre of praise and blame. The genre typically deals with the present. Bonnie Dow also points to the function of epideictic rhetoric, particularly when dealing with a crisis response, to "allow the audience to reach a communal understanding of the events which have occurred."[8] Particularly when making sense of the death of Americans, the President's epideictic discourse offers praise, blame, explains causes, and provides assurances for the events that make up the crisis. President Trump's speech is demonstrative of qualities of consummatory crisis discourse, which "is forensic because it attempts to present a case for the guilt"[9] of those responsible for the crisis. The speech is forensic, meaning there is a look back at the past for justification for actions and legal implications in particular. Trump states: "The best way—so important—and the best way to beat the drug crisis is to keep people from getting hooked on drugs to begin with."[10] This message hearkens back to the "just say no" rhetoric of the Reagan era of the war on drugs. Trump also touts ads and education, same as Nancy Reagan's "just say no" model, that will lead to a "drug-free generation of American children."[11] It neglects the complicated nature of addiction and underlying factors that could lead an individual to become involved with drugs and drug use. The Trump approach is, basically, a recycling of the failed Reagan approach. Michael McGrath poignantly notes of the former era's "just say no" approach as, "alarmist and damaging, a child-friendly arm of the continuing campaign to justify and perpetuate a 'war on drugs' with racially and economically disproportional targets."[12] This simplicity further lends itself to the criminal frame more so than a public health frame.

Denise Bostdorff argues that "what continues to make epideictic discourse an appealing rhetorical choice for political leaders is that it persuades on deliberative questions without seeming to do so."[13] Deliberative rhetoric is inherently persuasive and leads to decisions about what actions to take in the future. The deliberative genre of rhetoric is typically associated with political speeches, but as Bostdorff argues, epideictic rhetoric persuades without coming across to audiences as explicit persuasion. It also removes the debate and decision-making and rhetorically positions the policy approaches as foregone conclusions that a great and wonderful citizenry would naturally want and desire to see come to pass. The analysis that follows will demonstrate how Trump uses blame to further define the crisis as a threat to citizen safety, divisively political along party lines, a campaign opportunity, and, ultimately, solidifies his vision of the United States. Placing blame partially on the opposing party, that Trump will imply ultimately pushes the crisis further, and allowed it to be what it is before Trump declared the crisis a public health emergency.

The *War on Drugs* set a trend in the 1970s for how many presidential responses would follow. Joseph Gfroerer, statistician and supervisor of national drug surveys for the National Institute on Drug Abuse (NIDA) and the Substance Abuse and Mental Health Services (SAMHSA) writes, "Shortly after his announcement of the war on drugs, Nixon submitted legislation to Congress for consideration. The legislation emphasized interdiction, law enforcement, and the impact of drug use on crime more than public health. Under Nixon's proposed plan, primary federal responsibility and funding would fall under the Department of Justice."[14] There was, at its beginning, a large focus on the connection between drugs and criminality driving the need for understanding and writing new laws aimed at drug use in the United States. Law enforcement, since the beginning of the *War on Drugs,* has had a centralized role and the legal frame was firmly in place along with the metaphor of war. Surveys and data had been primed to focus upon the criminality rather than socioeconomic drivers for drug use since the beginning as well.[15]

There is a long-standing drug crisis in the United States. Since President Nixon declared the *War on Drugs* in the early 1970s, presidential speeches regarding the subject of drug use have followed fairly standard traditions and typical framing methods. Susan Mackey-Hallis and Dan Hahn found that "victimage rhetoric successfully offered guilt-relief to many Americans, defined and motivated a community by identifying common enemies, strengthened consent and marginalized dissent, created consensus about solutions, and weeded out corruption in the ranks by identifying those who were 'soft' on drugs."[16] Victimage is the process of redeeming guilt. Finding a place for blame is crucial and the legal frame is often the simplest in order to define and offer relief about something as complex as the opioid crisis.

This legal framing couched in terms of being "tough" or worse, being "soft," relates to a trend Mackey-Hallis and Hahn found and describe here: "From 1986 onward, the U.S. drug problem was often presented in discourse and specific actions in ways that were mutually supportive. The message was unmistakable: drug use in America was a national security issue."[17] The national security issue frame allows for a link to easily identifiable foes. Yartey argues "that securitization also concurrently diverts responses from civil society toward military and intelligence organizations that have the authority to outweigh the liberties of civil humanity."[18] Ultimately, Yartey finds that, while securitization metaphors and the use of terms like "combat" effectively garner support for responding to epidemics, they are also highly problematic and "viewing a disease as a national security threat to civil society."[19] These foes have appeared in Trump's speeches before and his base, who I will show is clearly in the immediate audience for the speech, can identify the trends of these foes' negative impacts upon the nation already.

The *war on drugs* in the United States has been fraught with racial inequities to say the least. Ashley P. Ferrell writes, "The intensive and by now well-documented 'war on drugs' and subsequent war on black and Latinx communities through the end of the twentieth century has had sustained consequences in major urban areas across the United States."[20] People of color often bear the brunt of the so-called "tough" policies that often land blame on the individual rather than addressing the historical and systemic issues that underlie drug use and dealing. There is also a stereotype that usually accompanies particular drug usage. Jeffery Chaichana Peterson, Aline Gubrium, and Alice Fiddian-Green found drug usage and crises are "stratified intersectionally by race, class, and gender. Analyses of U.S. popular culture illustrate the profoundly racialized nature of crack cocaine and the entrenchment of its perceived symbolic link to inner-city ghettos and People of Color"[21] while meth and the opioid epidemic in particular "has focused largely on the emergence of the White drug user as the face of this crisis."[22] A 2019 *PBS News Hour* report points out:

> The opioid epidemic in the United States has largely centered on white Americans, who account for roughly 80 percent of opioid overdose victims. But the national attention on white victims has pushed minorities to the sidelines, even as the number of opioid-related deaths among non-whites is on the rise.[23]

The report also points to the more systemic issues that would exclude communities of color from being part of the conversation, such as the history of the prior drug epidemics building mistrust between these communities and healthcare providers, less access to healthcare in general, and a litany of other healthcare-related inequities.[24] The epidemic was racially categorized as a "white" epidemic from the beginning. As public health experts F. D. Scutchfield and C. William Keck point out, deaths of despair—of which the opioid epidemic is the deadliest part of—is "a phenomenon first identified by Case and Deaton in a *Proceedings of the National Academy of Science* publication. Case and Deaton documented a rise in the mortality and morbidity of middle-aged White non-Hispanic men in the United States after 1998, but not in Hispanics or African Americans."[25] According to the *U.S. Census Quick Facts* website, New Hampshire is 93.1 percent white, like other states hardest hit by the opioid epidemic that have large percentages of their population made up similarly; such as West Virginia which is also 93.0 percent white.[26] It is not a stretch that disenfranchised white voters, commonly associated with Trump's base, would respond favorably and may not question some of Trump's fear tactics that include naming raced foes in the epidemic.

Racism is prominent in Trump's rhetoric and has been since his run for office in 2016. Critics of Trump's communications have commonly found that the term "American" is a softly veiled euphemism for "white" and his *borrowed*[27] campaign slogan "make America great again," as Carole McGranahan explains, "a time when America was great and when one had the right to be racist and misogynist."[28] Unsurprisingly, simplistic presentations of other countries factor into explaining the cause of the epidemic. Fear is a common rhetorical tactic that had been practiced by Trump since his presidential run and was built into his policy stances about building a wall and banning Muslims.[29] These fear appeals combined with the ethnocentric appeals lend itself to appealing to Trump's base, who is clearly present in the audience. At one point during the speech, part of the crowd chants, "Build that wall! Build that wall! Build that wall!" as Trump discusses how vital the wall on the southern border will be to stopping the epidemic.[30] Mexico and China are two external foes explicitly named throughout the speech as finding loopholes in current laws, streaming illicit drugs into our country, and feeding the crisis. These countries are deemed threats and engaged in illegal activities. If these foes are involved, it is not a leap for citizens to view their security, both nationally and individually, at risk.

LEGAL FRAME FOR THE OPIOID CRISIS

The legal frame is introduced early on in the speech. President Trump begins his speech in the typical way, standard of most political speeches, in that he offers praise to those physically present around him, including his wife Melania and the state of New Hampshire itself. He even recalls that the room where he is giving the speech is where he came for his first primary. Trump then moves into thanking Governor Sununu and a few other notable guests who will later be revealed as instrumental in the plans for ending the crisis: "I want to thank also Attorney General Sessions, and Secretary—thank you, Jeff. Secretary Azar, Secretary Nielsen, and Surgeon General Adams for joining us at this very important event."[31] Jeff Sessions was the Attorney General at the time, Secretary Azar was the Secretary of Health and Human Services, and Secretary Nielsen was the Secretary of Homeland Security. Nearly all of those thanked in this segment have responsibilities within the legal and national security realm. Only Secretary Azar stands out from this list as being the head of Health and Human Services. This is important to start out the speech with because it begins a long pattern of speaking about the crisis within a legal frame. The legal frame compliments the epideictic tone in a fascinating way. It effectively reinforces and bolsters the sites for blame the President assigns. Furthermore, it demands those that President Trump deems praiseworthy be in key positions of focus for ending the opioid crisis. By establishing the legal frame early, Trump is priming his audience for a legal and law-centered solution to the crisis.

Law enforcement specifically marked by the President orients the overall stance of the crisis and solutions that must follow the legal framing. The legal frame demands criminality solutions. The law enforcement cited is a synecdoche for the larger approach that he wishes to bring to the matter.

Shrouded in praise, the rhetorical maneuver of praising law enforcement and positioning the crisis as security threat is actually a deliberative position, yet the epideictic shroud hides this as an option—rather than a foregone conclusion—from the public for how to approach the crisis. Law enforcement on the state and federal level is thanked shortly after to build upon the different layers of the legal framing that Trump builds over the course of the speech. He began with the federal level and extends that further when he expresses his love for law enforcement: "We're also joined by a number of law enforcement officers who we love. Our police, DEA, ICE, Border Patrol agents, and Customs officers work night and day to keep drugs out of our communities and criminals off of our streets. So today, we thank you, we honor you, and we want you to know that we will always have your backs 100 percent. Thank you very much, law enforcement. Thank you."[32] Drugs and criminals are cited as the problem in this early statement and law enforcement is the obvious solution. Their efforts are cited as working towards the solution and Trump even remarks that his administration will support them "100 percent." Locating the issue on the streets and as a drug problem limits the possible solutions significantly and shines light on the ways in which Trump is defining the problem.

Praise for specific actions follows this list of law enforcement agencies shortly after they are named and their efforts are generally thanked by the President. By putting these actions at the beginning of the speech, the legal frame is further driven forward and the value of law enforcement efforts is prioritized. It also rhetorically forecloses debate about which approaches would be most advantageous given the sheer complexity of the opioid crisis. Here Trump describes some of the merit-worthy actions of law enforcement: "Our Customs and Border Protection—and these people, the job they do is incredible—seized nearly 1,500 pounds of fentanyl last year, nearly three times the amount seized in 2016. And I told China: Don't send it. And I told Mexico: Don't send it. Don't send it."[33] Customs and Border Protection being praised also blames outside forces for the opioid crisis and reinforces the synecdochal threat from outside of our borders. The epideictic function of blame places the insecurity of the nation due to this issue on familiar foes. China and Mexico are explicitly called out and blamed in this statement.

Key to epideictic rhetoric is the bivalent quality of simultaneous praise and blame. Praising the Customs and Border Protection agency is simultaneously blaming those they are enforcing against. China and Mexico are specified as sources of blame for sending drugs into the United States. These also coincide with some of the policies that Trump campaigned on and are clear nods to his promises to be tough on immigration and building a wall along the southwest border of the United States. Trump even praises the Immigration and Customs Enforcement's actions, or ICE, specifically when he states: "In

2017, ICE arrested criminal aliens with 76,000 charges and convictions for dangerous drug crimes."[34] The "dangerous drug crimes" arrests is vague, but through the purpose and context of the speech, it could easily be assumed those are being implied to be directly tied to the opioid crisis efforts.

New Hampshire, though a hard-hit state, is identified as doing things well through their criminal justice system. In the process of praising the state, Trump identifies the medical profession as partly to blame for the crisis. Trump offers praise in the form of statistics and evidence of their criminal justice system working hard to stymie the tide of the crisis: "Last year, the Department of Justice prosecuted more than 3,000 defendants in cases involving opioid, all of the trafficking, and the related crimes—3,000 cases—including a pharmacist, a physician's assistant, and an opioid trafficker, each charged with committing serious drug crimes in New Hampshire." Pharmacists, a physician's assistant, and an opioid trafficker are put side-by-side as equals in the blame category. These representative anecdotes that Trump lists visualizes the pharmacist and physician's assistant in a white lab coat as the drug dealer working alongside the already known criminal—the drug trafficker. This metaphorically places them as the same and demands the same type of legal approach—criminal punishment. Trump reinforces this message with this statement: "Whether you are a dealer or doctor or trafficker or a manufacturer, if you break the law and illegally peddle these deadly poisons, we will find you, we will arrest you, and we will hold you accountable. Thank you."[35] No one, not even those in white lab coats, are above the law in Trump's vision of the crisis. Doctors are not usually placed on the same level as drug traffickers, but Trump makes it clear that they are, and their culpability in the epidemic is the same. This amplifies and bolsters the legal framing of the epidemic and, in some ways, obfuscates the medicalization of the issue. It is not a public health issue, in spite of Trump declaring it a public health emergency the year before, it is a criminal issue. Even the doctors are subject to the same blame and penalties, though not all doctors writing prescriptions are doing anything illegal. Trump is praising New Hampshire's legal frame with this specific praise and the number of cases sounds impressive for a single year. There is no baseline established for what a typical amount of cases regarding opioids before the crisis would be for comparison, but the message of praise comes through clearly.

Equally important to the number of cases in this example of the legal frame is the way Trump's speech rhetorically levels drug dealers from the streets to pharmacies to doctor's offices as all being the same. The legal framing of dealing "deadly poisons" is firm within the first eleven minutes of the speech. Drug dealing and crime are familiar to the audience as going hand-in-hand. The medical professionals are new to this equation, but are consistently placed side-by-side with the familiar criminal trope. The response *should* involve law enforcement and criminal charges *ought to* be brought. The epideictic qualities of what easily could and perhaps should be a deliberative topic are consistently foreclosed in the speech. Trump continues with his praise of New Hampshire law enforcement and their justice system and concludes it by citing a particular operation, Granite Shield:

> Here in New Hampshire, I applaud all of the Drug Enforcement Agents and law enforcement officers who recently coordinated Operation Granite Shield, an 18-hour enforcement action targeting drug traffickers that resulted in the arrest of 151 people. These are terrible people, and we have to get tough on those people, because we can have all the Blue Ribbon committees we want, but if we don't get tough on the drug dealers, we're wasting our time. Just remember that. We're wasting our time. And that toughness includes the death penalty.[36]

The specification of the death penalty is essential and a theme that continues throughout the rest of the speech. Trump's "toughness" about the opioid crisis is put into clear terms and demonstrates the values placed on the criminal justice system. It also is a synecdoche borrowed from the approaches of administrations past and the familiar rhetoric of the "war on drugs." Casualties and death are expected in war, so the metaphor allows for and even excuses this level of action be taken. The death penalty is typically a divisive topic in the United States, but Trump uses it here as a way to express his commitment and express values that his base will surely identify with. His vision of the crisis demands this response and approach to the crisis. Accountability and blame for the crisis are firmly assigned within the first 15 minutes of the speech. The scales of justice weighing the crisis as a criminal issue is a clear extension of the war on drugs from decades past. The legal frame is front and center, which incorporates clear praise and accolades to law enforcement as well as a prescription for the solution: toughness on criminals, tightening our borders, and creating fear.

Trump's assessment of how the criminal justice system had been handling drugs before his initiatives were in place is glib and, of course, oversimplified. He blames how the system used to be, prior to his administration and handling of the crisis, for the problem. This implies blame be assigned to the Obama administration and praise for his. Through "toughness," his administration will induce enough fear that people will stop committing crimes. Here Trump explains:

> You know, it's an amazing thing. Some of these drug dealers will kill thousands of people during their lifetime—thousands of people—and destroy many more lives than that. But they will kill thousands of people during their lifetime, and they'll get caught and they'll get 30 days in jail. Or they'll go away for a year,

> or they'll be fined. And yet, if you kill one person, you get the death penalty or you go to jail for life.[37]

The toughness prescribed includes the death penalty for peddling poison. Drug dealers are coded as murderers with this statement. Murder is one of the few crimes that allots for the punishment of the death penalty to be assigned. This also simplifies the crisis vast complexities of the opioid crisis down to a crime metaphor. There are bad guys—the drug dealers and traffickers, victims—the users of opioids, and good guys—members of law enforcement—in this simplified vision of the crisis. It gives a more fully developed picture of the values in Trump's America. Drug dealers are killers and killers deserve the death penalty. The simplification lays in the assumption that the legal system works to put killers to death on a consistent basis and is a synecdoche of the justice system. A highly problematic one at best that could be incredibly divisive, but the immediate audience seems to be on board throughout. Trump continues to drive this point as he states: "So if we're not going to get tough on the drug dealers who kills thousands of people and destroy so many people's lives, we are just doing the wrong thing. We have got to get tough. This isn't about nice anymore." Praise is assigned to being tough and blame is put upon the prior administration for being "nice" to drug dealers and effectively not utilizing the criminal justice system to its full and ultimate potential of the death penalty.

Campaigning messages come out in this speech that further drive the epideictic sentiment of praise and blame. The current America, with Trump in the Oval office, is the most praiseworthy and valued America in this speech. He is the only one with the proper vision of the crisis to end it. Trump drives this point through not so subtle jabs that implicate the blame of the prior administration. Trump explains to the audience, "This isn't about committees. This isn't about let's get everybody and have dinners, and let's have everybody go to a Blue Ribbon committee and everybody gets a medal for, frankly, talking and doing nothing. This is about winning a very, very tough problem." The implications are abundant in this statement. Blame is implied and placed upon the prior administration for "talking and doing nothing" about the opioid crisis. Praise is assigned to the virtue and quality of Trump's "tough" administration. The "very, very tough problem" of the opioid crisis requires a tough on crime solution. Trump's administration has brought about and enabled this toughness that has allowed law enforcement as well as the criminal justice system to do what they do best. The value is placed on treating the crisis as a criminal one. Praising law enforcement explicitly emphasizes the need for legal solutions and criminal ramifications in order to stop the crisis. The paradigm of winning and losing is interesting here and does not necessarily fit within the legal frame. It gives a nod to Trump's additional purpose of the speech, which comes across as a campaign speech for a second term from time to time, and is explicitly seen here. Here Trump's campaigning mode comes across clearly: "I don't want to leave at the end of seven years and have this problem, okay? I don't want that. Right? Thank you. Not going to happen. Thank you all. A lot of voters in this room. I see that. Thank you."[38] A second term would be the ultimate praise and win that Trump is asserting he deserves with his particular brand of action and commitment to the opioid crisis.

Blame is not just particular to the prior administration. Trump assigns blame to the Democrats as a whole and does so by attacking their values. Doing nothing, keeping the borders open for the flow of opioids, and prioritizing things like DACA are all to blame as faulty values on the part of the opposing party. These are the values that Trump sees as antithetical to solving the opioid crisis. Trump extols the values and virtues that Americans ought to prioritize in order to end the crisis, which include: cutting off the supply of illicit drugs, border security, a wall to keep those drugs out. "The second part of our initiative is to reduce the supply of illicit drugs. Ninety percent of the heroin in America comes from our southern border, where, eventually, the Democrats will agree with us and we'll build the wall to keep the damn drugs out."[39] The first part of the initiative is to educate the public about the dangers of drug addiction. Trump asserts that his administration will be fiscally responsible about how to go about this education and, through a series of anti-drug commercials and a website where people can share their stories about the dangers of addiction, no one will want to do drugs anymore. The audience quickly responds with shouts of "Build that wall! Build that wall! Build that wall!" in support of the President's assertion that the wall is part of the solution to the opioid crisis. Trump also toes the party line of fiscal conservativeness by stating, "We're also going to make sure that virtually all prescriptions reimbursed by the federal government follow best practices for prescribing. We'll ensure that opioid addiction is not subsidized by the American taxpayer."[40] This is another campaign pitch moment in the speech. It is partially medical, the federal government will only support best practices for prescribing drugs, and ensures the taxpayer and the voters in the audience that they will not be taxed for solutions to the crisis that reached this point due to flawed policies and inactions of the Democrats.

Values and priorities are further praised and blamed after the audience shouts, "Build the wall!" Trump reinforces the flawed values and vision of America that the Democrats are putting ahead of doing something about the opioid crisis. The picture Trump paints is a glib one of inaction on the part of the Democrats. Their values are not to keep American citizens safe, but to prioritize immigrants who are contributing to the opioid crisis. The Democrats values of keeping the border open are allowing for the flow of heroin into our country. Here he proclaims praise for the Republican party, who is capable of prioritizing the opioid crisis and DACA simultaneously:

> The Republicans are totally in favor of doing something substantial for DACA. But the Democrats like it as a campaign issue, so they don't get it approved. And they want to tie it to the wall, which is okay with me. But both should get approved. They don't want it to be approved. Remember what I said: They don't want it to be approved. They want to make it part of the campaign. Well, we'll make it part of the campaign, also. And we'll win, because we're going to win on those issues.[41]

Trump's assertion here clearly spells out that the Democrats are in the wrong within the context of many things, but most pointedly within the context of this speech, the opioid crisis. Ironically, in a clear moment of him campaigning for a second term, Trump identifies the Democrats as blame-worthy for tying important issues to campaign leverage. The Democrats values are flawed because they are putting immigrants before citizens and Trump implies their values are allowing the flow of heroin into our country.

FEAR-DRIVEN SOLUTIONS

Anti-drug campaigns are part of the proposed solution, but it comes at an odd point in the speech, and is ultimately couched in between stronger, more developed points about law enforcement and legal solutions. Trump describes the "best" way to keep the problem from occurring in the first place here, "The best way—so important—and the best way to beat the drug crisis is to keep people from getting hooked on drugs to begin with."[42] This point demonstrates the tenuous rhetoric of the speech well. Prevention is a common strategy from public health experts and fits within the public health frame. Scutchfield and Keck argue that prevention will be vital to stopping the opioid epidemic and that "public health is now tasked with developing an approach to the primary prevention and management of opioid use and addiction in this vulnerable population."[43]

Trump furthers the point about prevention with details about how to keep people from getting hooked through the development of anti-drug commercials, "And this has been something that I've been very strongly in favor of: spending a lot of money on great commercials showing how bad it is, so that kids seeing those commercials during the right shows on television or wherever—the Internet—when they see these commercials they—'I don't want any part of it.'"[44] The President then compares these proposed commercials to the anti-smoking commercials and he assigns success to those. Ergo, the logic being, these anti-drug commercials will be successful. Even better yet, they will be fiscally responsible. He further explains, "That's the least expensive thing we can do, where you scare them from ending up like the people in the commercials. And we'll make them very, very bad commercials. We'll make them pretty unsavory situations." The toughness approach is still present in this portion of the speech. It breaks briefly from a criminal to and educational approach, but the implication is that you will die from the drugs or be put to death in these commercials that illustrate "pretty unsavory situations" you may end up in if you use drugs.

This is one of the few places where medicalization of the crisis briefly breaks the legal frame, but it still maintains the toughness and fear messaging, which is central to the legal, crime-centric solutions proposed before and after this small portion of the speech. Medicalization is the process of categorizing something in society as a medical issue. Antonio Maturo states, "the process by which some aspects of human life come to be considered as medical problems."[45] The medicalization becomes apparent when Trump uses the term *epidemic* instead of *crisis*. Trump states "This epidemic can affect anyone, and that's why we want to educate everyone."[46] The "very bad" commercials will ultimately scare people into not using drugs. Fear is viewed and valued as an educational tool in this discourse of the opioid crisis. The security metaphor takes on the level of personal safety in this brief portion of the speech. In order to keep oneself safe, it can be inferred, these approaches the crisis must be in place. Here, Trump uses the word "epidemic" instead of "crisis." The word "crisis" appears fourteen times in the speech and is complementary to the legal frame. The word "epidemic" only appears twice and is more complementary to the medicalization of the issue as it denotes disease. Crisis is more associated with challenges writ broadly and is not tied to disease, which better fits a medical-solution and framing of the issue as a whole. While the terms "opioid epidemic" and "opioid crisis" can be used interchangeably, it strikes me as a strategic maneuver, and crisis is a well-selected term to stick with for Trump's purposes. Putting the issues in terms of a "crisis" rhetorically bolsters the legal frame and criminal-centric solution to the problem. It also fits with the securitization and enables the blame upon doctors to be more comfortable than medicalization. Charging those same foes who helped create the problem, drug dealers in lab coats, with the solution would only add more to the tenuous treatment of the crisis in the speech.

DEATH PENALTY SOLUTIONS FOR A DEADLY CRISIS

Loopholes in laws and open borders are a consistent site of blame in Trump's speech. Getting those closed, adding new laws, and strengthening punishments all firmly reinforce the legal framing of the crisis. One loophole is online access into the country to sell drugs like fentanyl. Trump describes current efforts that have already partially been implemented to a degree of demonstrated success:

> We're also shutting down illegal online marketplaces and preventing drugs that come from China and other countries from bypassing our borders. And we're getting very tough on it. It's not that we have a choice. We don't have a choice. We can be nice, and we can be soft and weak, and you're not going to have a country left. So, we have to strengthen up, and strengthen up our laws so that we can do what we have to do. We have to stop this from happening.[47]

Many virtue-laden words are used in this brief statement. Being "tough" is a virtue. Being "nice," "soft," and "weak," perhaps how the prior administration was doing things will result in losing the country entirely. The words "tough," "toughness," and "tougher" are repeated twenty times in the speech. In this statement, China is clearly part of the blame for the opioid crisis with their selling of drugs over the Internet through "illegal online marketplaces," as well as other countries that are left unnamed. It is considered illegal to bypass borders through illegal methods, so this representative anecdote bolsters the legal framing of the crisis. Closing online loopholes is part of the new laws Trump proposes along with a myriad of others. The main focus of the laws is to lead to the ultimate consequence: the death penalty.

The death penalty is a strong theme and proposed solution to the opioid crisis throughout the speech. It comes up by name eight times and is alluded to several other times. Trump offers his rationale and evidence in a few places in the speech, but it comes through most explicitly when he vaguely references other leaders who implement the death penalty. Trump pulls this idea from other countries to support his claim that the death penalty is a fitting punishment for the criminality involved with the opioid crisis. This is an intriguing value to put forward as central to the solution in the United States. Trump offers up, without using specific country or leader names, an example of the dialogue he has had with other leaders who do not have drug problems. This portion of the speech is where he focuses on justifying implementing the death penalty:

> If you look at—if you look at other countries—I've gotten to know the leaders of many countries. And I won't mention names, but you know the countries I'm talking about. I go around, "How is your drug problem?" "We don't have much of a drug problem." "What do you mean you don't have a drug problem?" "Well, we don't have." I say, how come? "We have zero tolerance for drug dealers." I said, "What does that mean?" "That means we have the death penalty for drug dealers. We don't have a drug problem."[48]

Trump's example of dialogue with other countries' leaders offers insights into his reasoning and supports it by offering a nonspecific model of using the death penalty to eliminate drug problems as a whole in the United States. It works to his advantage to leave out specifics and fill them in. As is suggested by the audience chanting, "build the wall, build the wall" earlier in the speech, the immediate audience in the room can be trusted to follow this lead from Trump, they will pick up on the desired implications, and come to conclusions that Trump would want them to arrive at. The reasoning is simple, other countries that do not have drug problems implement the death penalty. Therefore, the United States should do the same.

While the epideictic genre functions to foreclose debate through emphasizing praise and blame for the present status of America, the President takes a moment to recognize one of the more controversial realities in his vision of the crisis. Trump yields momentarily in the speech and takes a few lines to recognize that the death penalty solution may not be a widely shared as a value of the rest of the country outside of the room. Here Trump concedes, "But the ultimate penalty has to be the death penalty. Now, maybe our country is not ready for that. It's possible—it's possible that our country is not ready for that. And I can understand it, maybe." Trump says it is "possible" but he does not concede that this lack of readiness is the present reality for the United States. He ends on the word "maybe." Trump continues his statement by nodding to his base, who is likely to agree with him, through asserting his personal belief and stance, "Although, personally, I can't understand that. But there are people that are good people, that are strong, smart people, and they would differ with most of us." When Trump asserts his belief and stance aligns with "most of us," he pivots into placing those who would disagree as a minority in the nation. He is praising the majority and blaming the minority who would hold up progress for ending the crisis because of their softness of crime. This also relegates and practically undoes the compliments of being "good," "strong," and "smart," because the minority who oppose the death penalty as part of the solution will simply be outvoted. Their virtues are rendered moot because they are the minority. Those in the minority, who do not support the death penalty, will be drowned out by better, stronger, and smarter people who want to end the crisis.

Trump argues that the majority of Americans are already behind the value of the death penalty, closing borders, and getting tough on the crisis. Trump affirms his values by concluding his recognition of those who may differ from his stance when he explains, "unless you have really, really powerful penalties, led by the death penalty for the really bad pushers and abusers, we are going to get nowhere. And I'm telling you, we are going to get somewhere."[49] Trump's values and the virtues of the death penalty being the leading punishment will prevail. This line of argument implies that these are indeed the present values and praiseworthy actions of the United States.

Tragedy and the death of loved ones are presented as the impetus for requiring such tough responses to the opioid crisis. The Mozer family who lost a child to opioid overdose is present at the speech and even speaks a bit. Botticelli and Barry cite:

> The use of a sympathetic narrative can also be an effective approach for stigma reduction. The use of narrative needs to be approached with some care given research showing that individual depictions can increase stigma by leading audiences to blame the affected individuals, as opposed to societal and other factors, for the problem they are experiencing.[50]

President Trump has them come up to the stage and hold a picture of their son. Trump introduces the couple and gives a bit of background about their son's path to addiction, "Here with us today are Jim and Jean Mozer. They lost their beautiful son, Adam, to a fentanyl overdose. His addiction began with prescription pills he found in their kitchen cabinet. They have since begun the Zero Left initiative to help families get rid of excess painkillers." Trump then apologizes to them for their loss, thanks them for their leadership and bravery, and welcomes Ms. Mozer up to the microphone to speak. She offers more about her son's character and concludes her story with this, "As smart as he was, he found his way into our kitchen cabinet. And, sadly, the rest is history. He got hooked on it, and had to go to the street eventually. And he found fentanyl."[51] The blame falls squarely on access to the drugs and most pointedly to the "streets" where he found the deadly and potent drug fentanyl. Fentanyl is one of the drugs that Trump has already called out other countries for bringing into the United States and further justifies his reasoning for closing borders. But as Botticelli and Barry point out, this contextualization right around the medicalized narrative of the sympathetic victim falling prey to mishandling of prescriptions and then deadly street drugs likely trafficked into the country may not be enough given the broader context of the legal framing pervasive throughout the speech.

The family does not operate solely as a synecdoche for the crisis, instead, the death of a son and their family tragedy act to rhetorically reinforce the need for stronger laws, more law enforcement, and shows the Nation what is at stake if these policies are not implemented. The Mozer family tragedy represents the heartfelt loss of one family and is extrapolated out to the rest of the nation. It also fits well with the securitization metaphor. Ms. Mozer finalizes her statement by ending on a highly emotional note, "And he's been gone for two-and-a-half years, and we miss him every day. Thank you."[52] It has become fairly standard in political speeches to include a family or individual whose story illustrates a broader point through a specific case. It is important that the family is from New Hampshire, where the speech is taking place, and is from a state that has been grappling with rates of death that are, as Trump describes in the first few minutes of the speech, "Every day, 116 Americans die from an opioid-related overdose. In New Hampshire, the overdose, really, death rate—I mean, can you believe this? The death rate is double the national average. It's got difficulties like people wouldn't believe."[53] The Mozer family illustrates this point and does not detract from Trump's legal framing of the issue. Their loss and their son work toward supporting the legal frame. The people pushing the drugs on the streets are to blame, not the victims whom fall prey to their nefarious, illegal deeds.

FOES, FAILURES, AND THE PRAISEWORTHY ONES

Trump's vision of the crisis is rather telling about his vision of America. This vision is revealed through how he constitutes the crisis. Naming foes, failures, and those worthy of praise constitutes and defines the crisis in particular terms. Getting "tough" will be the way out of the crisis. The legal framing of the crisis and emphasis upon law enforcement leads to inevitable conclusions that demand particular actions. Getting tough means more legal actions and police responses to foes involved in the crisis. Those actions include using the justice system rather than the health care system to respond. Or even repairing the broken health care system that is partially responsible for the opioid epidemic to begin with. Treating doctors as criminals, even the well-meaning ones who were duped by pharmaceutical companies, is part of the plan in Trump's vision. First responders are mentioned as praiseworthy, but only twice in the speech. This suggests that the legal frame does not yield as much focus on the medical side of the crisis.

Trump mentions first responders and lifesaving overdose-reversal drugs briefly in his speech. These measures are relegated to the third part of the administration's plan to end the crisis and yield to the medicalization of the crisis since it is a medication-centric solution. Medicalization shows up in the speech when it deals with the victims of the crimes of the foes identified. Here Trump explains briefly, "The third part of our initiative is to get lifesaving help to those who need it. We're going to make sure our first responders have access to lifesaving overdose-reversing drugs—which, by the way, are amazing."[54] Trump uses this opportunity in the speech to praise the innovation and charity of "Mike Kelly, the president of Adapt Pharma. Adapt Pharma makes an overdose-reversing drug for opioids, which I've watched and seen work. It's called Narcan. It's actually incredible. Today, we applaud Adapt Pharma's decision to provide free—free—Narcan to all high schools, colleges, and universities in America."[55] As a quick aside and as someone whose partner works in the public health field, I can personally attest that this part of the plan has not been delivered upon yet. Narcan is not readily provided to first responders across the nation for free. It is something that first responders must purchase or work with their local counties to get supplies of. Sometimes grants are available for the procurement, but those funds are limited and the grants are not always accessible to the first responders directly.

The legal framing of the crisis puts the crisis in more simple terms an audience can quickly identify with and understand better. Illegal activities are also something that law enforcement can deal with. It alleviates the pressure on the general public entirely. Everyone can continue their daily lives and be unencumbered by the death going on around them. The foes are explicitly named as drug dealers, doctors, drug traffickers, "peddlers of poison," China, and Mexico. Jeffery Chaichana Peterson, Aline Gubrium, and Alice Fiddian-Green argue "Criminal justice system officials benefit from drug problems . . . Punitive solutions are favored."[56] Trump, an outspoken supporter of law enforcement, supports law enforcement further by framing the issue in terms of criminality and downplaying the role of public health, even though he declared it a public health emergency. He then responded to health with criminality approaches. At best, his messaging is inconsistent and at worst, misleading about the true nature and complexity of a deadly issue.

The victimage cycle of redemption is set in motion by clearly identifying the crisis as due to criminal activity and easily identifiable foes. If you deal with the foes, crisis stops. Not really, but the criminality framing provides that rationale. Trump's vision of the crisis also strongly follows in the footsteps of Republican administrations before him by framing the current opioid issue as Nixon, Reagan, and George H.W. Bush did. Criminal activity and a threat to national security. China and Mexico are posing the most clearly identifiable national security risks. These risks further support Trump's vision of America that includes tighter borders and a wall along the southwest border to keep drugs from flowing in from Mexico. These also tie into some of Trump's other appeals to rally his base that included building a wall and stopping immigration.

Failures on the part of the Democrats and the prior administration are many. The blame for those failures that lead up to and allowed the crisis to reach such a deadly point is foisted upon the Democrats in several places in the speech. Trump lists: doing nothing, being soft, being nice, holding committee meetings and dinners, not pursuing stricter laws, the death penalty as a punishment, and closed borders are all failures mentioned explicitly. In exact opposition and in support of policies that he campaigned on in the same state of New Hampshire during his primaries, Trump is lists praiseworthy virtues that he demonstrates as: toughness, being active, supporting law enforcement, closing borders, reducing the supply of illicit drugs, changing policies for prescribing, and calling upon the justice system to declare the death penalty a suitable punishment for this deadly criminal activity driving the crisis. The epideictic function of praise and blame occurs simultaneously. Blame assigned to the Democrats simultaneously implies praise for the Republicans. Trump does not waste this moment to campaign for four more years at the helm.

Overall, the speech presents Trump an opportunity to define a crisis, campaign, and further develop his vision of making America great again. And parts of that vision are rather appealing. Toward the end of his speech, Trump states: "We will defeat this crisis, we will protect our beautiful children, and we will ensure that tomorrow is better, brighter, stronger, and greater than ever before. Because as long as we have trust in our citizens, pride in our country, and faith in our God, we will not fail."[57] This is a beautiful sentiment and it is something the entire nation can support. The epideictic sentiment is strong as Trump concludes the speech by praising and extolling the virtues of trust, pride, faith, and strength.

Though medicalization and the public health frame appear in this speech, it is haunted by the criminal-centric approaches held over from the rhetoric of the "war on drugs." The criminality and law frames override it entirely. Botticelli and Barry argue, "The historical overreliance on law enforcement approaches to address substance misuse, combined with discriminatory racial attitudes, led not only to incarceration of drug dealers and the pursuit of cartel leaders, but more consequentially to a large incarceration of low-level, nonviolent offenders arrested for simple possession or drug use."[58] Ultimately, securitization replaces medicalization. This is far and away from the other case studies. Even the HIDTA ODMAP, a law enforcement agency, frames the issue as an epidemic, not a crisis. HIDTA's ODMAP utilizes both public health and medicalization frames. Furthermore, the response is a blend of public health, medical, and behavioral responses that law enforcement agencies support. The oddity of the highest office at the federal level, who in part helps deem large allocations of funding to HIDTA, finding the crisis a criminality-centric issue is troubling to say the least.

Trump's response to the crisis and framing yielded little results. Reporting in an October 2020 *Vox* article, German Lopez cites, "Based on the preliminary federal data, drug overdose deaths spiked in 2019 to nearly 72,000. That was slightly higher than the previous record high for a single year in 2017."[59] Ultimately, the continuance of old and already proven to be ineffective legal approaches to the drug scourge Trump proclaimed would end under his watch actually got worse. The legal frame also encourages seeing people involved with drugs in a stigmatized light. Botticelli and Barry state:

> Misperceptions and lack of understanding of addiction as a chronic disease have promoted the criminalization of individuals with substance use disorder rather than a public health approach. The case is made for policy changes that support new policy directions that stress parity in treatment for mental health and substance misuse with other "physical health" conditions as well as suggestions for better communications strategies to reduce stigma.[60]

Trump's reliance upon the legal frame and obfuscating the public health or medicalization approach furthers stigmatization of drug users as well as those "peddling poisons," because users associate with criminals to get their drugs. It is too difficult to ask the general public to separate the two, particularly when things like MAT (medication-assisted treatment) are underfunded and widely unavailable for those who need help, and the criminality framing is so prominent at the highest level of governmental response to the issue.

Finally, the legal frame displaces the public health frame and demands traditional law enforcement approaches. Trump even goes so far as to punish with the death penalty as a fair and tough approach necessary to end the crisis. Willis and Painter cite the failings of prior approaches to end drug use in America here, "It is important to realize the implications of the 'war on drugs' and the effect such policies have had on drug use and addiction. The 'war on drugs' ultimately has been unsuccessful in reducing drug use in America."[61] The tenuous use of multiple frames in this speech demonstrates the tensions the opioid epidemic is rife with and helps with comprehending the enormous perceptual shift required. Having any medicalization and the public health frame present directly conflicts with approaches that are crime-centric and do not account for a complete picture of the underlying causes. Continuing with old rhetoric of the prior administrations, that did not prevail in drug use reduction throughout America, but did reinforce damaging stigma about individuals who use drugs, is detrimental to the progress needed to end the epidemic.

NOTES

1. "Ending America's Opioid Crisis," *Whitehouse.gov,* 2020, https://www.whitehouse.gov/opioids/.

2. "March 19, 2018: Remarks on Combating the Opioid Crisis," UVA Miller Center, 2019, https://millercenter.org/the-presidency/presidential-speeches/march-19-2018-remarks-combating-opioid-crisis.

3. Ibid.

4. Kate Snow, "Trump to Roll out Opioid Plan Monday, Including Tougher Punishment," *NBC News,* March 15, 2018, https://www.nbcnews.com/politics/donald-trump/trump-roll-out-opioid-plan-monday-including-tougher-punishment-n857141.

5. Ibid.
6. "Ending America's Opioid Crisis," *Whitehouse.gov,* 2020, https://www.whitehouse.gov/opioids/.
7. Ibid.
8. Bonnie J. Dow, "The Function of Epideictic and Deliberative Strategies in Presidential Crisis Rhetoric," *Western Journal of Speech Communication*, 53(Summer), (1989): 296.
9. Ibid, 297.
10. "March 19, 2018: Remarks on Combating the Opioid Crisis," UVA Miller Center, 2019, https://millercenter.org/the-presidency/presidential-speeches/march-19-2018-remarks-combating-opioid-crisis.
11. Ibid.
12. Michael McGrath, "Nancy Reagan and the Negative Impact of the 'Just Say No' Anti-Drug Campaign," *The Guardian,* March 8, 2016, https://www.theguardian.com/society/2016/mar/08/nancy-reagan-drugs-just-say-no-dare-program-opioid-epidemic.
13. Denise M. Bostdorff, "Epideictic Rhetoric in the Service of War: George W. Bush on Iraq and the 60th Anniversary of the Victory over Japan," *Communication Monographs,* 78 (3), (2011): 297.
14. Joseph Gfroerer, *War Stories from the Drug Survey: How Culture, Politics, and Statistics Shaped the National Survey on Drug Use and Health* (Cambridge: Cambridge University Press, 2019), 13.
15. Ibid, 14.
16. Susan Mackey-Kallis and Dan Hahn, "Who's to Blame for America's Drug Problem?: The Search for Scapegoats in the 'War on Drugs,'" *Communication Quarterly,* 42 (1), (1994): 6.
17. Ibid, 6.
18. Franklin Nii Amankwah Yartey, "The Critical Condition of Rhetorical Choices," *Journal of International Communication* 21 (2), (2015): 234.
19. Ibid, 236.
20. Ashley P. Ferrell, "'Righting Past Wrongs': Rhetorical Disidentification and Historical Reference in Response to Philadelphia's Opioid Epidemic," *Rhetoric & Public Affairs* 22 (4), (2019): 550.
21. Jeffery Chaichana Peterson, Aline Gubrium, and Alice Fiddian-Green, "Meth Mouth, White Trash, and the Pseudo-Racialization of Methamphetamine Use in the U.S," *Health Communication* 34 (10), (2019): 1176.
22. Ibid., 1173.
23. Jenae Addison, "How Racial Inequity is Playing Out in the Opioid Crisis," *PBS News Hour*, July 18, 2019, https://www.pbs.org/newshour/health/how-racial-inequity-is-playing-out-in-the-opioid-crisis.
24. Ibid.
25. F. D. Scutchfield and C. William Keck, "Deaths of Despair: Why? What to do?," *American Journal of Public Health* 107 (10), (2017): 1564.
26. "Quick Facts: New Hampshire," United States Census Bureau, 2019, https://www.census.gov/quickfacts/fact/table/NH/PST045219.

27. I say *borrowed* here because the slogan was also used by President Ronald Reagan.

28. Carole McGranahan, "A Presidential Archive of Lies: Racism, Twitter, and a History of the Present," *International Journal of Communication* 13 (2019): 1374.

29. Joseph P. Zompetti, "Rhetorical Incivility in the Twittersphere: A Comparative Thematic Analysis of Clinton and Trump's Tweets During and After the 2016 Presidential Election," *Journal of Contemporary Rhetoric* 9 (1/2), (2019): 51.

30. "March 19, 2018: Remarks on Combating the Opioid Crisis," UVA Miller Center, 2019, https://millercenter.org/the-presidency/presidential-speeches/march-19-2018-remarks-combating-opioid-crisis.

31. Ibid.

32. Ibid.

33. Ibid.

34. Ibid.

35. Ibid.

36. Ibid.

37. Ibid.

38. Ibid.

39. Ibid.

40. Ibid.

41. Ibid.

42. Ibid.

43. F. D. Scutchfield and C. William Keck, "Deaths of Despair: Why? What to do?." *American Journal of Public Health* 107 (10), (2017): 1565.

44. "March 19, 2018: Remarks on Combating the Opioid Crisis," UVA Miller Center, 2019, https://millercenter.org/the-presidency/presidential-speeches/march-19-2018-remarks-combating-opioid-crisis.

45. Antonio Maturo, "Medicalization: Current Concept and Future Directions in a Bionic Society," *Mens Sana Monographs* 10 (1), (2012): 122.

46. Ibid.

47. Ibid.

48. Ibid.

49. Ibid.

50. Michael Botticelli and Colleen L. Barry, "Stigma and the Language of Addiction." In *A Public Health Guide to Ending the Opioid Epidemic*, edited by Jay C. Butler, and Michael R. Fraser (Oxford: Oxford University Press, 2019), 41.

51. "March 19, 2018: Remarks on Combating the Opioid Crisis," UVA Miller Center, 2019, https://millercenter.org/the-presidency/presidential-speeches/march-19-2018-remarks-combating-opioid-crisis.

52. Ibid.

53. Ibid.

54. Ibid.

55. Ibid.

56. Jeffery Chaichana Peterson, Aline Gubrium, and Alice Fiddian-Green, "Meth Mouth, White Trash, and the Pseudo-Racialization of Methamphetamine Use in the U.S," *Health Communication* 34 (10), (2019): 1175.

57. Ibid.

58. Michael Botticelli and Colleen L. Barry, "Stigma and the Language of Addiction." In *A Public Health Guide to Ending the Opioid Epidemic*, edited by Jay C. Butler, and Michael R. Fraser (Oxford: Oxford University Press, 2019), 35.

59. German Lopez, "Trump Said the Opioid Epidemic Would Go Away. It Didn't," *Vox,* October 20, 2020, https://www.vox.com/future-perfect/21522973/trump-biden-opioid-epidemic-drug-overdoses-addiction-election-2020.

60. Michael Botticelli and Colleen L. Barry, "Stigma and the Language of Addiction." In *A Public Health Guide to Ending the Opioid Epidemic*, edited by Jay C. Butler, and Michael R. Fraser (Oxford: Oxford University Press, 2019), 32.

61. Erin Willis and Chad Painter, "The Needle and the Damage Done: Framing the Heroin Epidemic in the Cincinnati Enquirer," *Health Communication* 34 (6), (2019): 668.

Chapter 5

Mapping the Epidemic

ODMAP and the Boundaries of Response

Robbie Gonzalez, science and technology writer for *WIRED,* begins his article talking about blame. "Big pharma," "cheap pain pills and cheaper heroin," and even our "mesolimbic reward system" in the brain are called out as potential sites for this blame. Gonzalez's call to action was simple, "Just don't wallow in it—the blame. Wallowing takes time, and with opioid abuse killing close to 100 Americans a day, time is in exceedingly short supply."[1] The answer to speed up the response to the opioid epidemic, in part, comes through technology. Mapping technology, more specifically. A real time, collaborative map accessible to government agencies—most of which are law enforcement and first responders—that assists with coordinating agencies across the country, nuancing their responses, and equipping life-saving countermeasures to sites of opioid overdoses.

The Overdose Detection Mapping Application Program, or ODMAP, created by the Washington/Baltimore High Intensity Drug Trafficking agency (W/B HIDTA) is a tool created by the federal government. Jeff Beeson, Deputy Director of the W/B HIDTA, defines the tool as, "an overdose mapping tool that allows first responders to log an overdose in real time into a centralized database. This tool allows us to capture all fatal and nonfatal overdose incidents on a shared data platform across agencies and across the country."[2] A resource accessible across agencies anywhere in the nation may not seem like much, but the exigence created by the opioid epidemic spurred this progressive undertaking. Beeson, as quoted in the *WIRED* article states, "We've never had overdose data like this before—and we've never shared it with each other."[3] The "we" Besson refers to are law enforcement, first responder, public health agencies, as well as state and federal government agencies. With the opioid epidemic raging, innovations such as ODMAP were cultivated and implemented to alert areas to anticipate overdoses and be prepared with naloxone, an opioid overdose-reversing medicine.

ODMAP and the ODMAP site offers an interesting case study for exploring the rhetorical dimensions of the opioid epidemic and government response. According to the program, ODMAP is "a product of the Washington/Baltimore High Intensity Drug Trafficking Area (W/B HIDTA)."[4] The map "offers the ability to collect both suspected fatal and nonfatal overdoses, in real time, across jurisdictions, to mobilize a cohesive and collaborative response."[5] Furthermore, ODMAP responds to the exigence of a lack. A lack in the government's response to the opioid epidemic to track, collect data, and respond. Visualization of overdoses provides a unique tool for the government to utilize in order to respond. ODMAP is available to governmental agencies across the country. Since 2017, its success is measured in its use as well as measures made easier to implement based upon the data the tool provides. By autumn 2020, ODMAP had "logged more than 335,000 suspected overdoses submitted by nearly 30,000 users."[6] Examples of measures implemented that save lives and reduce the number of overdoses include: drug takebacks, public education, peer recovery outreach, and understanding where spikes are occurring to the measures are implemented in the right spots within a community.[7] Agencies that use ODMAP have data at their fingertips and ways to see trends in nearby counties to better anticipate overdose spikes.

Communication across agencies across the entire country, not just situated in a single-state, and the simple visualization are the most poignant features that sets it apart from other apps. The ability to communicate between participating agencies and share data is an enormous achievement and success that intersects public safety and public health agencies where there had been a lack before the tool was created. The ODMAP website features an additional map titled "ODMAP Overview: Washington | Baltimore HIDTA," which is an esri Story Map.[8] The ODMAP Overview map, which I will refer to as the Overview map for clarity henceforth, is part of the community-oriented argument to join this nation-wide collaboration in the fight against the opioid epidemic. ODMAP launched January 2017, initially as a three-county pilot in West Virginia,[9] and is now present in nearly every state in 2019.

In this chapter, I explore the rhetorical dynamics of ODMAP, Overview map, and the exigence from which it is a product of. Visualization is a powerful modality. Visualization of the detection and response is a key feature of the rhetoric of the opioid epidemic. If we can see it, it follows that we can detect it and respond to the epidemic accordingly. Arguing for the tool's effectiveness and gaining as many users as possible is also essential for the technology to operate to its full potential. Brightly color-coded circles on a gray colored map of the United States shine like beacons of both despair and hope that the governmental response can make change and start to reverse the savage trends of death the opioid epidemic has wrought. My objective in this chapter is to trace how this visualization operates in the broader topography and visual synecdoche of the opioid epidemic. More specifically in this chapter, at the federal-level of governmental response. I also seek to articulate the governmental vernacular of the epidemic. The public health frame and medicalization are prominent throughout the map and site promoting its use. This chapter explores the terms used, operational definitions, what the responses are, and how visuals and language interact. I explore the context for the content in the ODMAP site, analyze the visualizations, and finally discuss how ODMAP functions rhetorically to define the opioid epidemic and responses to it. First, a brief theoretical review for how I will be regarding maps as rhetorical and sites of important production of terms, definitions, and strategy.

MAPS AS VISUAL RHETORIC

Tracking disease and epidemics through maps has been practiced for centuries. They function, in part, to concretize abstract concepts and simplify complex sociopolitical landscapes. Maps portray a space, stabilize the complexities of space and time, and provide authority.[10] Maps are not necessarily seen as arguments, but rather, objective artifacts that represent a place. Timothy Barney asserts that, "cartography is a rhetorical process."[11] Barney articulates the rhetorical potency and politics of a map well when he states, "a confluence of social forces that constrains a culture's sense of its space and its place within it."[12] Related to that point, Michel De Certeau argues that maps act as "interlocutors" with the context and content they are created out of. Maps are formed and informed by narratives and the social discourse surrounding them.[13] By marking and informing the boundaries of the visual information being told, maps are interlocutors that aid the authority of the rhetor. The rhetors for ODMAP are participating agencies and HIDTA. This story of epidemic is informed and formed by the players highlighted in the map. The narratives and the maps provided are concomitantly providing boundaries of response, information, and evidence of success of response.

As "living mediums," maps are constrained and enabled by the audience and the context in which they are read and processed as evidence. Maps are evidence of the present, which is represented in real time in this case, and the future. According to Candice A. Welhausen, "[maps] tell us what is possible to know and believe about the future, which in turn allows us to have some sense of power, authority, and ultimately control over that future."[14] This is complementary to the public health framing and medicalization of the epidemic. Treating it like the epidemics that have come before, this mapping technology concretizes the medicalization of the opioid epidemic in enticing and effective visual ways. Participation mediums, like the collaborative space of the ODMAP, rely upon user-participation in order to be useful and effective communication tools. Maps functions as *evidence* and simultaneously are persuasive. The evidence from the map depends upon participation and gathering as much data as possible. There is the underlying assumption that if you can map it, it can be predictable, and there must be an exigence demanding its use. Through the impartiality and objective perspective commonly associated with the medium, maps are often not viewed as rhetorical or even capable of parsing and stabilizing a dynamic space.[15]

Visuals hold enormous power to persuade. Cara Finnegan points to the vital nature of understanding the role of visuals in contemporary society. The ways in which visual rhetoric "governs and authorizes" is of particular interest for this chapter.[16] Lawrence Prelli finds rhetorics of display, such as maps, are prolific in our society. Furthermore, rhetorics of display participate in discourse as sites of "epideictic rhetoric" which is key because it "commands members of a community to join together" and the work of proof is already completed in the visual demonstration.[17] The community of public safety and public health are put into a community with the common goal of reducing the epidemic through data and sharing of that data. Through the call to share data and empower the community through its usage, ODMAP calls on law enforcement, public health officials, and health responders into a community. The more the community utilizes the tool, the more robust and effective their responses can be. It is easy to forget that visuals make arguments and constrain the view of something. Maps imbue the featured area with qualities from other modes of communication and concretize information in an objective manner. Additionally, they visually compress large amounts of information into comprehensible data that is processed quickly by the brain. Maps ground and place information in an analyzable form that allows for assessment. In this case, a specific response.

Times of transition and the use of technologies, such as a collaborative mapping application program, demonstrate the invention of the rhetorical situation. The best means of persuasion come out of these moments when communication is vital to curbing the epidemic and literally saving lives. Amber Davisson remarks, "Isolating rhetorical texts produced during these time periods can offer rich insight into how rhetorical invention takes place in moments of change, how media users and consumers adapt to changes in technology, and how these transitions are interpreted in larger social discourses."[18] ODMAP is such an instance that demonstrates the rhetorical inventions afoot during the ongoing opioid epidemic well. Joining the first responder community across the nation in real time is expressed as vital by the ODMAP site. The "larger social discourses" of the opioid epidemic surely demanded an approach to remedy it from first responders, public health officials and agencies, and an inventive use of technology came out from that demand.

Maps effectively constrain situations as well as responses to situations. They offer a snapshot of a situation and are easily digestible visually. Karin Wilkins describes maps as a way to make sense of complex sociopolitical or geopolitical dynamics.[19] The map can bring something abstract, such as an epidemic and the horrors of opioid overdose, to a familiar and concise form of expression. The map simplifies complexities and puts information into an easy to read format. Maps establish a frame and create a space that is then imbued with information. The information embedded in them is presented as a *way of viewing* something strategically. ODMAP is a tool for governmental, health, and first responder agencies. It has also crafted arguments about what the opioid epidemic is and is continuing to define and mobilize responses to it.

EXIGENCE OF THE EPIDEMIC

Epidemics and maps to visualize them are not novel. The Center for Disease Control (CDC) uses maps or "Geographic Information System Data (GIS)" as a tool on a regular basis. There is an entire chapter in their manual titled: *The CDC Field Epidemiology Manual.*[20] However, the CDC typically tracks diseases that are not tied to a substance abuse disorder. And the response is typically not one that involves a detailed collaboration of law enforcement, first responders, as well as public health officials. What is novel about ODMAP as a tool is tri-fold. First, it is a collaborative tool that is accessible to any government agency across the country. Second, ODMAP works in real time and also tracks nonfatal overdoses. Finally, it is a centralized database and reduces the time it was taking to understand trends and anticipate where overdose spikes will occur next. To emphasize the lag in this process and the uniqueness of ODMAP, Gonzalez remarks of the power of the tool saying, "understanding where and how people are overdosing can take local health and law enforcement months to suss out."[21] Tracking overdoses in real time, going across state and county lines, coordinating data from multiple agencies, and working across multiple government agencies make ODMAP a standout technology in the fight against the opioid epidemic.

Deaths of despair have been occurring since 1998. Around that time, life expectancy began to decrease for middle-aged, non-Hispanic whites, without a college degree. This is the first-time life expectancy has decreased for the aforementioned demographic in the United States. Overdose and suicide surpassed cancer and heart disease as the leading causes of death in the United States since the turn of the twenty-first century. Economists Anne Case and

Angus Deaton, who coined the term *deaths of despair,* state, "the prescription of opioids for chronic pain added fuel to the flames, making the epidemic much worse than it otherwise would have been."[22] Case and Deaton also found the group, in addition to decreasing life expectancy, reports an increase of chronic pain.[23] Not surprisingly, the opioid overdose portion became a top priority for federal government agencies to attend to and develop novel approaches to. But the approaches did not have to be novel and the rhetoric drastically shifted away from the "war on drugs" of the past, that emphasized and demanded high-incarceration rates, and were ultimately useless for decreasing drug use. Here, with ODMAP, HIDTA—in spite of being a drug trafficking deterrent and generally law enforcement-centric agency—has adopted the public health frame and medicalized narratives to endorse their new, Naloxone-centric approach. The bodies of those experiencing an opioid overdose—the deadliest portion of deaths of despair—and their response to doses of Naloxone are the focus of the map and priority of the agencies involved.

W/B HIDTA Deputy Director Jeff Beeson sums up the exigence for ODMAP here, "In 2016, 63,600 overdose deaths were reported across the country, a dramatic rise from the 52,000 deaths in 2015. Despite these dramatic statistics, the country lacks a consistent methodology to track overdoses, which limits our ability to understand and mobilize against the crisis."[24] In 2018, Jeff Beeson cites the statistic of "overdose death tolls of 115 Americans every day."[25] Clearly the response needs more work. ODMAP is part of that work. Since it is a tool that relies heavily on crowd-sourcing, I analyze the ODMAP site overall as an argument and method of persuasion. The site itself is persuasive and a way to attract more agencies to utilize the tool and join the community of public safety and public health facing the epidemic head-on. Specifically, the Overview map is an argument and rhetorically-potent site of persuasion to garner agency participation. As of September 2020, there are "3,300 participating agencies in 49 states, the District of Columbia, and Puerto Rico.[26] The call to join in participation is being heard. The call is simple, "This tool is only available to government (state, local, federal, or tribal) agencies serving the interests of public safety and health."[27] Also, compelling and specific to whom will participate in this particular community the map needs to participate in order to be an effective tool to mitigate the opioid epidemic.

MAPPING THE OPIOID EPIDEMIC AND RESPONSE

The initiative of W/B HIDTA's ODMAP is important to note: "Reducing overdose deaths by supporting statewide adoption of ODMAP and strengthening the ability of communities to leverage the data to develop coordinated public safety, public health, and behavioral health intervention strategies."[28] A few facets of the initiative stand out. The success of the tool, ODMAP, is correlate to reduction of overdose deaths. Statewide adoption of the technology is arranged as the first order of business for W/B HIDTA. The second is the "strengthening communities" in order to have a multitier response. Organizing data in order to organize and successfully deploy resources is the function of the mapping tool. The overview map assists with the argument that all agencies eligible ought to participate and utilize ODMAP. I will cover the overview map in the next section. Participation in the technology is key realizing a decrease in overdose deaths related to the opioid epidemic. Coordinating public safety, public health, and behavioral health is the final and most novel portion of what the tool brings to the fight. It is also the most rhetorically fascinating because it reorients and reinforces the power of using the term "epidemic." Naming and responding to the epidemic as such make it clear that it is not a drug-issue. Rather, it is a health issue that requires participation and care from all aforementioned communities in the W/B HIDTA ODMAP initiative.

At a glance, ODMAP appears similar to other maps used to track epidemics. The W/B HIDTA states their aim with the ODMAP visual interface is to "focus on temporal and spatial patters using overdose data analysis to: track as a disease, assess changes in patterns and behaviors, [and] respond with actionable intelligence."[29] The map interface is fairly straightforward. The map appears, at first, as a tool. A centralized data repository. The technology is simple and straightforward by design. ODMAP enforces and reinforces the parameters of the epidemic and codifies the response to it simultaneously. Locating and anticipating where the epidemic will intensify is part of the parameter set. The map assists with detecting and predicting the movement of particular batches of opioids so more resources may be deployed and officials may be alerted by ODMAP that an intensification of overdose is headed their way. Another key feature of the map is to track the successes of the response: Naloxone. Success and failure are defined as whether or not the overdose resulted in death. If Naloxone reversed the overdose, the parameter implies it a successful interaction. The next step is to connect the overdose survivor with behavioral health resources. Naloxone and behavioral health involvement cooperate with the term epidemic in a rhetorically-potent way to reinforce the public health approach and medicalization of the issue.

The aesthetics of the map itself are telling. The United States is a dark gray with white boundaries. Bright colors atop neutral gray visually reinforce a "deviation" from the norm.[30] The deviation, in this instance, is the disease of opioid addiction. These data points visualize where life-saving medications, such as Naloxone, are needed most. The medicalized narrative is visualized through the brightly colored data points on the map. It can also be indicative of particular batches of opioids that are more potent, therefore driving an increase in overdoses once an area is hit. Nearby counties, for example, receive notifications of overdose spikes and observe protocols to enhance their response. Gray is the *standard* area which makes the bright colors stand out even more than they would against a white background. Names of states and a few major cities rest atop the gray in white, sans serif font. A "powered by esri" logo is situated at the lower right corner of the map.

The map is centered in the screen and the largest portion of the visual focus. The level 2 user may zoom into particular areas or have a view of the entire nation. Welhausen remarks, "in Western cultures, in particular, the placement of visual information creates a hierarchy, conveying the level of importance of each design element."[31] On the upper-left of the dashboard, a legend, just as you would expect to find on a regular map. The legend is titled "Suspected Overdoses." The legend below the title classifies the symbols and colors appearing on the map to the right. Diamonds denote a fatality. In the United States, the diamond symbol typically denotes a hazard. A red diamond means "Fatal: No Naloxone." A yellow diamond means "Fatal: Single Dose Naloxone." A green diamond means "Fatal: Multiple Doses Naloxone." Colored circles are "nonfatal" overdoses. A teal circle means "Non-Fatal: No Naloxone." A green circle means "Non-Fatal: Single Dose Naloxone." A purple circle means "Non-Fatal: Multiple Does Naloxone." A white circle means "Non-Fatal: Naloxone Unknown." A white square means "Unknown." The colors correspond with the Level 1 user's codes for entering information to ODMAP while they are responding to an overdose. Their application has a color-coded menu that they simply click the appropriate color-code for what occurred on the call through their mobile device. Contrast is a key visual component. The bright colors and white text represent the hope that using ODMAP to "better combat the opioid epidemic."[32]

The user can adjust the data through drop-down menus. On the left, the "Total Suspected Overdoses" gives a number from the prior twenty-four hours if there are no other filters set. The sample visual provided on the ODMAP.org site rests at a count of 8,704 "suspected overdoses" in the last twenty-four hours. This provides an argument in itself. It also posits the rhetorical question: what would this number be if more agencies were actively reporting? Below that the total is split between "fatal" and "Naloxone." This is an interesting way to divide the numbers when the legend suggests that there are fatal overdoses even when Naloxone is given. On the right, under "Suspected Overdoses," the drop-down menu options filter by state, countries, incident date and time by date range and quarter, fatal, and Naloxone administered. Naloxone is featured in most sections of the ODMAP interface. The user is bound to preset measurements provided by the W/B HIDTA creator of the tool. As well as the argument that Naloxone is central to the response to the epidemic.

At first glance, ODMAP is a tool for law enforcement, first responders, and public health officials. More than a tool, it provides an important visual framework for participating agencies. Davisson argues "the combination of visual language, statistical data, and cartographic representation" as a powerful one.[33] ODMAP is not simply a tool or centralized data repository. It is an argument about the opioid epidemic, what the response ought to be, and a community building tool. It affirms and argues that Naloxone is central to reducing the epidemic. Therein lies an argument about and reinforcement of the medicalization of the issue. ODMAP is an important symbol and visual expression of the opioid epidemic. Naloxone is an intersect that binds the public safety and public health communities further by being complementary to both the public safety and public health sides of the epidemic. It is a medical response that affirms both parts of the community through its use, distribution, and being a tool that keeps people alive to receive an intersectional response from facets of health, behavioral, and law agencies. These approaches combined include things to assist those who survive an overdose by connecting them with physicians, behavioral health experts, and law enforcement assisted diversion or LEAD.[34] This gets survivors the medical and behavioral help the need and keeps them out of jail or prison, which may not be helpful at all. By 2017, Naloxone and other overdose-reversing drugs had been identified part of the federal government's strategy to "combat the Opioid Crisis."[35]

ODMAP: AN EPIDEICTIC COMMUNITY BUILDING TOOL

The ODMAP produces a visual argument and hails a particular community to action. The community brought together under the common cause, the soaring rate of death in the opioid epidemic. Furthermore, the overview map uses mapping to persuade that mapping is essential to fighting the epidemic. The use of a particular response, administration of Naloxone, is a key facet of the ways in which public safety and public health agencies can impact the epidemic across the country. Beeson cites that "most American jurisdictions do not share data among law enforcement, fire departments, and emergency medical services, and even fewer do so in real time. ODMAP eliminates this data-sharing dearth by centralizing all agencies' data relating to overdoses within one platform," which leaves a community of people on the frontlines of the epidemic disparate.[36] ODMAP calls for them to cooperate and collaborate in one place.

The ODMAP site offers a robust, dynamic, and interactive place for the community to converse and find resources. Beeson describes it as "which will include an online repository for materials developed by users, a webinar series sharing promising practices, and a monthly newsletter to share updates. The goal of the ODMAP User Community is to facilitate the sharing of materials, practices, and ideas among ODMAP users."[37] Trainings, seminars, and support are all available on the site, which keeps users returning to the site to upload data and increase their ability to respond to the epidemic. The overview map contains multiple arguments to support the participation and effectiveness of the ODMAP tool.

OVERVIEW MAP: A STORY MAP

The overview map is a rich, dense, and visually stimulating text. It is an esri Story Map and features visuals, videos, and text boxes throughout. An overview map that chronicles the history of the ODMAP tool is what the site purports the purpose to be. The description of the story map instructs: "Scroll through the presentation below to see how ODMAP began its journey, how it has grown, and where it is headed with this visual overview."[38] The purpose of the map is actually two-fold. The overview story map chronicles the history of ODMAP, but also more importantly, functions to persuade and attract potential users to ODMAP. It operates as an argument for new users and an argument to existing users of the power, potential, and need for the tool. Additionally, the map reifies and concretizes the community ODMAP has formed.

Just after the site prompts vendors to collaborate, the overview map appears next. A sweeping aerial visual that covers the bustling metropolitan Washington D.C. area directly around the nation's capital building. In the foreground, centered against the moving background, is a text box that reads, "ODMAP Overview: Washington | Baltimore HIDTA."[39] The visual overview map is interactive. The user scrolls through at their pace, read informational text boxes, click for additional information from resources outside of the overview map, and view embedded videos as they peruse the map. The overview map covers a lot of territory. Once the user begins to scroll down to interact with the map, a menu across the upper right of the menu appears with the following navigation button options: Home, The Concept, The History of

ODMAP, Continued Growth, Statewide Usage, Applying the Data, Success Stories, and Future of ODMAP.

The *story* of the epidemic is laid out in a compelling way through this interactive map. The menu across the top allows the user to easily move to the portions of the map desired or most useful for their interest in adopting the ODMAP technology. The menu invites exploration of the map and is highly visual synecdoche of the medicalization of the epidemic. Interactivity itself is a rhetorical device. According to Barbara Warnick and David S. Heineman, "Online interactivity, therefore, functions as a means of activating user responses and as a mode of address that can influence users and can itself be rhetorical in its effects."[40] The overview map is a mode of address to a particular audience: agencies whom can collaborate and are directly involved in the governmental response to the epidemic. In spite of the sheer volume of information, the map flows well and is easy to get through large portions of it in a relatively short amount of time. Perhaps most effective is the inclusion of success stories and testimony from actual users of ODMAP.

What the opioid epidemic *is* comes into view shortly after entering the overview map interface. The first section of the story map is titled "Home." Under the heading, "Addressing the Problem," the exigence of the opioid epidemic is explained in terms of opioid overdose deaths and the key demographic for turning the tide of the epidemic: nonfatal overdose victims. Non-fatal overdose victims become a locus point of the overview map as well as ODMAP. The story map explains, "Non-fatal overdose victims constitute a high priority group and a logical point of intervention to reduce overdose mortality rates."[41] This will directly connect to ODMAP user testimony featured further into the map. The use of the term "victim" is rhetorically rich in itself and reinforces the disease model under the broader expression of *epidemic.* The main audience for the ODMAP technology and site in general is law enforcement, first responders, and public health officials. All of whom are charged to protect and serve the public. The term *victims* connote an individual who is harmed or injured as a result of a crime, accident, or other event. It removes the agency from the victim and enhances the need for action from the community called forth to respond to the epidemic. Victims also need the assistance and help of law enforcement, first responders, public health officials. This rhetorical choice forecloses criminality or punitive responses. Removal of agency from the victim reduces the suggestion of criminality and displaces blame away from the individual whom experiences overdose. The disease model and medicalization of this discourse reinforces the action suggested in the ODMAP: overdose reversal, Naloxone implementation, connecting victims with behavioral health resources, and focusing on saving lives.

The biomedical model, public health frame, and medicalization are evident immediately in the map. The biomedical model of medicine focuses on disease and upon the biological failing of systems within the body.[42] Textually, information derived from the CDC are used to support the exigence of the epidemic and affirms the medicalization of the issue. "Overdose deaths in the United State continue to rise, from 63,632 in 2016 (Centers for Disease Control and Prevention [CDC], 2017) to 70,237 in 2017 (CDC, 2018)."[43] Death is the ultimate failing of systems of the body and opioids are the mechanism for the failure. Law enforcement and first responders collaborate on several issues with the assistance of the CDC. While these types of collaborations are not novel, it is still rhetorically important. CDC is charged with investigating and researching health issues. Therefore, beginning the map and defining the epidemic with terminology and data from the CDC defines the epidemic in terms of health, not crime. The lack of technology is set up in the overview map along with the definition of the problem. This is an absence that ODMAP fills. Further along in the "Addressing the Problem" section, the map explains;, "In order to effectively address the opioid and overdose epidemic, one centralized platform must be established for ease and timely communication and data sharing."[44] The problem and solution are spelled out clearly in the first section of the map.

Visuals are included that reinforce the medicalization of the issue and the specific role that law enforcement, first responders, and public health officials have. The overview story map bolsters the argument by using the same medium it is persuading its audience to utilize in order to more effectively fulfill their role in stymying the epidemic. Below data from the CDC, on the left, are images of lethal doses of heroin and fentanyl. The word "dose," commonly used in medical settings for prescriptions, is used here. The visual of a dose of both appear to the eye as small amounts. However, the lethal dose of fentanyl stands out more than the dose of heroin because there are only a few white flecks of fentanyl in the glass vial. Furthermore, Fentanyl is commonly associated with a medical context, as it is a prescription drug. Yet, it is more deadly in this particular context of the opioid epidemic. To the right of that image is a chart that demonstrates the "3 Waves of the Rise in Opioid Overdose Deaths."

The cartographic representation of data demonstrates and reinforces the biomedical model. The first wave begins with medically prescribed opioids causing overdose deaths. The biomedical model is focusing upon the failing of systems that cause pain, pain is treated without the larger consideration of the psychological and social context—or the patient's "life world," and is part of what lead to the epidemic.[45] Limited medical access is what is articulated as the push toward heroin in the second wave. There is a note below fentanyl and "other synthetic opioids" that these are "prescribed or illicitly manufactured."[46] The inclusion of the term prescribed reinforces the medical framing of the epidemic further. Each wave is medicalized in some manner. Welhausen cites, "statistical graphics are particularly powerful rhetorical constructions because they are simultaneously both visual and scientific forms of communication."[47] On top of the visual and scientific credibility, the user is invited to engage further and through the images, which are set up as hyperlinks. This invites interactivity and increases the engagement of the user with the interface.

The story map includes medicalization at every step of explaining ODMAP. This interpretation of the space is essential for understanding the intentions behind crafting the map. Welhausen also remarks that "the purpose of creating any map is to arrange select geographic content into an abstracted visual representation that emphasizes certain features and minimizes others (inclusion and exclusion) in constructing new spatial relationships that advance a particular understanding and interpretation of that space."[48] Inclusion of the medicalization frame is apparent throughout. Highlighting prescription opioids and synthetic opioids: Tramadol and Fentanyl. Heroin, while included and more likely to be associated with criminal behavior, contributes the least the opioid overdose deaths. It is diminished further as it is only included in the data for the second wave of the epidemic. Commonly prescribed opioids and synthetic opioids, particularly the latter, are accountable for the most deaths and are most relevant to efforts because they account for the third wave of the epidemic. The third, or current wave, of the epidemic is the main focus of ODMAP and of the overview map. These are also likely drugs that law enforcement and first responders have encountered while responding to calls. The particular audience for the story map can readily identify with these visuals from their professional experiences.

The inclusion of particular sources of information lend credibility to the ODMAP technology and the successful, voluntary adoption of the tool. The source of the image and graph come from law enforcement in a state hit hard by the epidemic. All of the sources used in the story map are from within organizations that are included in the ODMAP user community. Knowledge from fellow community members also impacted by the epidemic is vital for the credibility of the story map as well as a successful pitch for adopting ODMAP technology. According to Andrew Flanigan's recent study of interorganizational law enforcement communication practices, "Tacit knowledge is acquired only through shared experience."[49] Featuring "Success Stories" from law enforcement hit hard by the epidemic and utilizing ODMAP to change and enhance their response to the epidemic is essential for persuading new users to identify with the existing community and to join. New communication tools hinge upon credibility from fellow law enforcement and the integrity of the technical system itself. This new tool rhetorically affirms the medicalization and public health frame of its approach. It provides evidence and a tool to better end the epidemic simultaneously. As Flanigan remarks "successful implementation and use of these tools relies on high *trust*—of fellow officers."[50] The inclusion of data from a fellow organization with experience, expertise, and significant findings is crucial for the adoption of the ODMAP and reinforces the argument for the voluntary adoption of the technology.

Using ODMAP also furthers the common cause of the community through data. Data is pitched as vital to the response and rests the argument upon overdose reversals that save lives. Parameters for what qualifies as data are as follows: overdose reversals, fatal overdoses, and number of doses of Naloxone. Data from ODMAP has been demonstrated as effective for expanding legislation useful for combating the epidemic. It follows that participating agencies join the community on the right side of the response. More data, is inherently argued in the map, necessary for a more robust response to the opioid epidemic. It also argues that more data will give a more realistic picture of the epidemic itself. That will ultimately lead to a better response and reduction of the epidemic.

Fellow law enforcement officers are featured in the section titled, "Success Stories." Current users of the system are first-hand witnesses to the epidemic, are fighting the epidemic already, and can offer the most viable insights about how ODMAP is improving their efforts. Including users whom are successfully using the technology and seeing reductions in opioid overdose deaths is an effective inclusion for adoption of the technology itself and it works to reify the medicalization of the issue. The biomedical model and medicalization is reinforced due to the success being largely based upon the overdose reversal by use of a drug, Naloxone. The saving of the life, because of a medical intervention, is what allows for the rest of the success story to happen. It also puts the medicalization, the expertise and science of the medical approach, first in the order of what needs to happen for the success to occur.

The first example in the section is from Erie County, New York. The ODMAP is organized county by county throughout the United States. A YouTube video embedded in the map is of a news story covering the utilization of ODMAP. The broadcaster states, "ODMAP connects health officials with people who overdose." Already, the medical framing of the police officer's role in the epidemic is at the forefront of understanding the use of ODMAP and the epidemic. Captain Brian Gould of the Cheektowaga Police, the officer interviewed says, "We're not going to arrest our way out of this problem." This demonstrates the power in the shift of the discourse of the opioid epidemic and offers hope that there are effective methods for dealing with this public health crisis that break away from past endeavors that were focused on punitive measures as deterrents. Furthermore, Captain

Gould states the connection with a "peer navigator" is key to the solution after explaining their officers were often going to the same houses and seeing the same people over and over again. Dealing with the opioid epidemic with the assistance of ODMAP is a "perfect combination" of resources and getting coordinated health care officials connected to the overdose victims.[51] This framing puts police officers more into a medical role and a mediator role of connecting victims with health resources. Arrests, or treating the issue as a crime, is explicitly discounted in the interview. After the video, the user scrolls to additional information in a text box that further explains:

> The Erie County Health Department utilizes ODMAP as a tool to identify treatment referrals. Health Department staff members monitor ODMAP for new points throughout the county and interface with local police who provide a copy of the police report. The Health Department's Peer Recovery Specialists then go to the overdose victim's home with a police officer and discuss treatment options. In the first 90 days of this program, 47% of referrals remain connected to care after 30 days.[52]

This demonstrates for the user of the overview map what the process of using the technology of ODMAP will look and feel like. It also gives insights about the success of including ODMAP and the decrease of strain on police once the overdose victim is connected with health resources from the County Health Department. The story of the opioid epidemic is given a public health frame, medicalizes the issue by suggesting medical and behavioral health solutions, along with a narrative of health resources as the solution. Naloxone being a life-saving medication and one of the initial treatments to reverse overdose and ultimately, rob the disease of victims.

The overview map discusses data in the section titled, "Applying the Data."[53] Representative examples of how ODMAP has been utilized by existing users start off the section. The emphasis of partnerships, with ODMAP as a tool as the central node, is repeated throughout the section. These partnerships are between eligible users of ODMAP: law enforcement, first responders, and public health officials are present in the example. A suggestion after partnerships is the utilization of "National Density Analysis." This example demonstrates how the partnerships grow with increased participation and data placed in the ODMAP database. The text reads, "armed with the information and data that ODMAP can provide, partners and analysts will be able to equip decision makers with the tools they need to create data-driven solutions to the opioid crisis."[54] As the user scrolls, the story map zooms in to give a more detailed look at the powerful "national density hotspot" capabilities that ODMAP supports. Visuals always work in tandem with the argument the text makes in the overview map. Data visualizations are provided to bridge any possible cognitive gaps. It also assists with the familiarity of the ODMAP system and reinforces tropes from disease maps. Welhausen's research of disease maps yields that, "disease maps visually reinforce the biomedical model through specific etiology by mapping single variables of interest," the variable being reversal of overdoses through the deployment of Naloxone in this case.[55] Naloxone is one part of the picture on the map and overall strategic response of many of the participating agencies. What is visually left out and visually silent are the other components of the response—the implementation of peer support, behavioral health experts, diversion, etc.—thereby the biomedical model and medicalization win out the argument in the visual of the map.

NALOXONE: THE MEDICALIZATION OF RESPONSE

Each entry into ODMAP is centered upon one key facet: was Naloxone used? If so, how many doses? Naloxone is a rescue medication given to someone suspected to be in the thralls of an opioid overdose. It is an overdose-reversal drug that blocks the receptors, displacing the opioid, and allowing time for first responders to get the individual to a hospital for medical care. Naloxone is a medication carried by many first responders, law enforcement, and is becoming more prevalent in everyday situations. Narcan, a nasal spray version of Naloxone, is now offered at many pharmacies and can be found in retail store and library first aid kits. The emphasis on naloxone codifies it as a response to the epidemic. Second of the five "specific strategies that H[ealth and] H[uman] S[ervices] will bring to the fight," from the *U.S. Department of Health and Human Services* is "promoting use of overdose-reversing drugs."[56]

The emphasis upon an overdose-reversing medication, Naloxone more specifically, is an interesting argument considering the source and authority behind the map, W/B HIDTA. HIDTA, or the High Intensity Drug Trafficking Areas program, was created by Congress in the late 1980s along with the Anti-Drug Abuse Act of 1988. By the mid-1990s, the purpose of the HIDTA programs was "to reduce drug trafficking and production the United States."[57] This demonstrates the rhetorical influences and social discourses surrounding the implementation and design behind the ODMAP. By the 2017 launch of the tool, the focus of the epidemic set upon preventing overdose deaths and providing addiction treatment. Partnering law enforcement with first responders and public health agencies was paramount to the success of combating the epidemic. Tom Carr, W/B HIDTA Executive Director, makes clear in a presentation to introduce ODMAP, "treating those who are ill—we recognize drug use disorder as a disease of the brain and body, NOT a moral failure."[58] The focus is a disease and the opioid issue is tracked as a disease on a map.

It is different from a choropleth map that visualizes areas in various colors and looks like a heat map. Choropleth maps had been used by HIDTA before to focus on areas of violence and conflict as it pertained to drugs, mostly illicit. Here, with the ODMAP, a medication is central to the response. Not arrest. Not the perpetrators. Instead, the victims of overdose. The variables are implementation of Naloxone and either the success or failure of the overdose reversal. Referring public health officials to the higher user levels of the map in order to connect the overdose patients to more resources is highlighted on the ODMAP website in the "Spike Response Framework" section. The first step is to "Connect: Interdisciplinary OD Response Team" to the affected area.[59]

The individuals impacted are actually missing from the map itself. For data security purposes, information about the individual is not part of ODMAP. The data rests on the following variables: location, fatal or nonfatal, whether or not Naloxone was administered, and how many doses. As part of the initial introduction of ODMAP, Carr references esri's memorial map of loved ones lost to the opioid epidemic as part of the impetus to do better fighting the epidemic. The argument for ODMAP rests upon the loss of human life and supports the medical perspective. *Celebrating Lost Loved Ones to the Opioid Epidemic* is another collaborative map that is open to the public and relies on participation of those who have lost a loved one to the epidemic. Photos and as much information as the user who posts wants to provide are the content for that map.[60] It provides a more human perspective on the exigence for ODMAP.

An absence of human presence and those individualized details in ODMAP assists with the objectivity of the medical lens to the epidemic. It comes across as more objective and data-driven. Cartographic visuals and maps are commonly identified as scientific, which often leaves humanity and morality out of the frame. Data becomes the focus and the map function as a medical response is clearly the focus. The social discourse surrounding the map covers the human element of the epidemic. In the overview map, the user has the option to click a hyperlink and learn more about the different types of opioids, perhaps types they have yet to encounter in the area they serve. The terms *epidemic* and *victims* are reinforced through data and general mission to serve the public with progressive medical and public health-centric approaches. Interactivity engages the user in the overview map—interactivity being a compelling mode of persuasive address—hails a particular audience, invites them to join the ODMAP community, and offers additional resources to better the fight against the opioid epidemic. The map itself is a synecdoche of the whole epidemic that offers a beacon of hope to those directly charged with turning the tide of the epidemic.

NOTES

1. Robbie Gonzalez, "This App Maps Opioid Overdoses in Real Time: Opioid Overdoses Proliferate, Like a Disease. A New App Lets Health and Law Enforcement Officials Anticipate their Spread," *WIRED,* September 22, 2017, https://www.wired.com/story/baltimore-built-an-app-to-map-opioid-overdoses-in-real-time/.

2. Jeff Beeson, "ODMAP: A Digital Tool to Track and Analyze Overdoses," *National Institute of Justice,* May 14, 2018, https://nij.ojp.gov/topics/articles/odmap-digital-tool-track-and-analyze-overdoses.

3. Robbie Gonzalez, "This App Maps Opioid Overdoses in Real Time: Opioid Overdoses Proliferate, Like a Disease. A New App Lets Health and Law Enforcement Officials Anticipate their Spread," *WIRED,* September 22, 2017, https://www.wired.com/story/baltimore-built-an-app-to-map-opioid-overdoses-in-real-time/.

4. "Home," *ODMAP.org,* 2019, http://odmap.org/#home.

5. Ibid.

6. Aliese Alter and Mitch Cunningham, "Where Public Health and Public Safety Intersect," *Sheriff & Deputy* 73 (1), (2020): 45.

7. Ibid, 46.

8. Ibid.

9. Jeff Beeson,"ODMAP: A Digital Tool to Track and Analyze Overdoses," *National Institute of Justice, May 14, 2018,* https://nij.ojp.gov/topics/articles/odmap-digital-tool-track-and-analyze-overdoses.

10. Candice A. Welhausen, "Power and Authority in Disease Maps: Visualizing Medical Cartography Through Yellow Fever Mapping," *Journal of Business and Technical Communication* 29(3), (2015): 261.

11. Timothy Barney, """'Gulag'—Slavery, Inc.": The Power of Place and the Rhetorical Life of a Cold War Map," *Rhetoric & Public Affairs* 16 (2), (2013): 321.

12. Ibid, 324.

13. Certeau, M. d., *The Practice of Everyday Life* (Berkeley: University of California Press, 1984), 122.

14. Candice A. Welhausen, "Power and Authority in Disease Maps: Visualizing Medical Cartography Through Yellow Fever Mapping," *Journal of Business and Technical Communication* 29(3), (2015): 279.

15. Timothy Barney, """'Gulag'—Slavery, Inc.": The Power of Place and the Rhetorical Life of a Cold War Map," *Rhetoric & Public Affairs* 16 (2), (2013): 325.

16. Lester C. Olson, Cara A. Finnegan, and Diane S. Hope, "Introduction." In *Visual Rhetoric: A Reader in Communication and American Culture*, edited by Lester C. Olson, Cara A. Finnegan, and Diane S. Hope (Thousand Oaks, CA: Sage, 2008), 1.

17. Lawrence Prelli, *Rhetorics of Display* (Columbia, South Carolina: University of South Carolina Press, 2006) 3.

18. Amber Davisson, "Beyond the Borders of Red and Blue States: Google Maps as a Site of Rhetorical Invention in the 2008 Presidential Election," *Rhetoric and Public Affairs* 14 (1), (2011): 119.

19. Karin Wilkins, "Mapping Fear and Danger in Global Space," *International Communication Gazette* 71 (7), (2009): 561.

20. Stephanie Foster, Erica Adams, Ian Dunn, and Andrew Dent, "Geographic Information System Data: Epidemic Intelligence Service," *Centers for Disease Control,* December 13, 2018, https://www.cdc.gov/eis/field-epi-manual/chapters/GIS-data.html.

21. Robbie Gonzalez, "This App Maps Opioid Overdoses in Real Time: Opioid Overdoses Proliferate, Like a Disease. A New App Lets Health and Law Enforcement Officials Anticipate their Spread," *WIRED,* September 22, 2017, https://www.wired.com/story/baltimore-built-an-app-to-map-opioid-overdoses-in-real-time/.

22. Anne Case and Angus Deaton, "Mortality and Morbidity in the 21st Century," *Brookings Papers on Economic Activity* (Spring 2017): 399.

23. Ibid, 400.

24. Jeff Beeson, "ODMAP: A Digital Tool to Track and Analyze Overdoses," *National Institute of Justice,* May 14, 2018, https://nij.ojp.gov/topics/articles/odmap-digital-tool-track-and-analyze-overdoses.

25. Ibid.

26. Aliese Alter and Mitch Cunningham, "Where Public Health and Public Safety Intersect," *Sheriff & Deputy* 73 (1), (2020): 45.

27. "Home," *ODMAP.org,* 2019, http://odmap.org/#home.

28. "The ODMAP Initiative," *Comprehensive Opioid Abuse Program,* 2019, https://odmap.coapresources.org.

29. Tom Carr, "Fighting the Opioid Epidemic with ODMAP," *Washington/Baltimore High Intensity Drug Trafficking Area,* Spring 2017, http://proceedings.esri.com/library/userconf/nss17/papers/nss_02.pdf.

30. Candice A. Welhausen, "Power and Authority in Disease Maps: Visualizing Medical Cartography Through Yellow Fever Mapping," *Journal of Business and Technical Communication* 29(3), (2015): 275.

31. Ibid, 265.

32. "ODMAP Implementation Examples," *ODMAP.org,* 2019, http://odmap.org/#home.

33. Amber Davisson, "Beyond the Borders of Red and Blue States: Google Maps as a Site of Rhetorical Invention in the 2008 Presidential Election," *Rhetoric and Public Affairs*, 14 (1), (2011): 107.

34. Aliese Alter and Mitch Cunningham, "Where Public Health and Public Safety Intersect," *Sheriff & Deputy* 73 (1), (2020): 46.

35. "5-Point Strategy to Combat the Opioid Crisis," *U.S. Department of Health and Human Services,* August 7, 2018, https://www.hhs.gov/opioids/about-the-epidemic/hhs-response/index.html.

36. Jeff Beeson, "ODMAP: A Digital Tool to Track and Analyze Overdoses," *National Institute of Justice,* May 14, 2018, https://nij.ojp.gov/topics/articles/odmap-digital-tool-track-and-analyze-overdoses.

37. Ibid.

38. "ODMAP Overview," *ODMAP.org,* 2019, http://odmap.org/#home.

39. Ibid.

40. Barbara Warnick and David Heineman, *Rhetoric Online: The Politics of New Media* (New York: Peter Lang, 2012), 53.

41. "ODMAP Overview," *ODMAP.org,* 2019, http://odmap.org/#home.

42. Albert Farre and Tim Rapley, "The New Old (and Old New) Medical Model: Four Decades Navigating the Biomedical and Psychosocial Understandings of Health and Illness," *Healthcare* 5 (4), (2017): 88.

43. "ODMAP Overview," *ODMAP.org,* 2019, http://odmap.org/#home.

44. Ibid.

45. Albert Farre and Tim Rapley, "The New Old (and Old New) Medical Model: Four Decades Navigating the Biomedical and Psychosocial Understandings of Health and Illness," *Healthcare 5* (4), (2017): 89.

46. Ibid.

47. Candice A. Welhausen, "Power and Authority in Disease Maps: Visualizing Medical Cartography Through Yellow Fever Mapping," *Journal of Business and Technical Communication* 29 (3), (2015): 269.

48. Ibid, 268.

49. Andrew J. Flanigan, "The Impact of Contemporary Communication and Information Technologies on Police Organizations." In *Law Enforcement, Communication, and Community*, edited by Giles, Howard (Philadelphia, PA: John Benjamins Publishing Company, 2002), 85–105.

50. Ibid, 99.

51. "ODMAP Overview," *ODMAP.org,* 2019, http://odmap.org/#home.

52. Ibid.

53. Ibid.

54. Ibid.

55. Candice A. Welhausen, "Power and Authority in Disease Maps: Visualizing Medical Cartography Through Yellow Fever Mapping," *Journal of Business and Technical Communication* 29 (3), (2015): 271.

56. Thomas E. Price, "Secretary Price Announces HHS Strategy for Fighting Opioid Crisis," *National Rx Drug Abuse and Heroin Summit,* April 19, 2017, https://www.hhs.gov/about/leadership/secretary/speeches/2017-speeches/secretary-price-announces-hhs-strategy-for-fighting-opioid-crisis/index.html.

57. "High Intensity Drug Trafficking Areas (HIDTAs)," *United States Drug Enforcement Administration, Department of Justice,* 2019, https://www.dea.gov/hidta.

58. Tom Carr, "Fighting the Opioid Epidemic with ODMAP," *Washington/Baltimore High Intensity Drug Trafficking Area,* Spring 2017, http://proceedings.esri.com/library/userconf/nss17/papers/nss_02.pdf.

59. "Spike Alerts," *ODMAP.org,* 2019, http://odmap.org/#home.

60. "Celebrating Lost Loved Ones," *esri,* 2019, https://opioidepidemic.maps.arcgis.com/apps/StoryMapCrowdsource/index.html?appid=19f5247b5bd043dda9a25b22c0919760

Chapter 6

A Brief Analysis and Sample of the Chronic Pain Management Debate in the United States

The debate about pain may strike some as surprising. Pain is pain, right? Not for the last decade. From defining pain, how people end up in pain, definitions of chronic pain, how to verify it, and whether or not people should have to experience it at all, let alone endure it for years, is all up for debate. This debate has been waging for the last decade. The issue about pain stems outward from the opioid epidemic. It is a contentious debate as well. Without pain, after all, we would not have the epidemic of opioid abuse and startling statistics of death. It seems people are willing to take opioids in order to avoid pain, doctors were more than willing to treat pain, and many are doing so at their and their patients' peril. Sometimes completely unwittingly. We live in a society and culture that generally views pain as negative, an impairment, and something to get rid of.[1] Numbing and treating with opioids came about in the early 1990s. Of course, the risks were not widely known.

Generally, the debate breaks down into two camps: either you are sympathetic to the patients experiencing pain and champion their right to access, or, you are more worried about the public health emergency that is the opioid epidemic.[2] Not to say these are the only voices present, but these are the loudest and most resounding sides of the debate. The pain management debate is typically about sufferers of chronic pain. Access to opioids for those patients is the access that most are concerned about. A few definitions may be in order. First, let's take the term chronic pain. Chronic pain, according to researchers Andrew Rosenblum, Lisa A. March, Herman Joseph, and Russell K. Portenoy, "has been described as pain that has persisted for at least 1 month following the usual healing time of an acute injury, pain that occurs in association with a nonhealing lesion, or pain that recurs frequently over a period of months."[3] Second term, opioids. "The term *opioid* refers to all compounds that bind to opiate receptors. Conventionally the term *opiate* can be used to describe those opioids that are alkaloids, derived from the opium poppy; these include morphine and codeine."[4] Synthetic opioids are what, according to the *Center for Disease Control,* describe as the "third wave" of the opioid epidemic that "began in 2013, with significant increases in overdose deaths involving synthetic opioids, particularly those involving illicitly manufactured fentanyl."[5] Fentanyl came to popular media attention in a notable way with the accidental overdose death of the artist Prince in 2016. The performer unwittingly was taking a medication that was laced with the powerful synthetic, fentanyl, and died at the age of fifty-seven. Tom Petty died of a fentanyl overdose the following year, which kicked off another round of media attention to these powerful drugs that doctors administer on a regular basis.

The debate sprawls from newspapers, to academic conferences and journals, the medical field as a whole, podcasts, blogs, and so on. I chose to focus on the past five years—2015 through 2020—of articles in *The New York Times, Time* magazine, and *NPR's All Things Considered.* Each did series and long-term reporting on the opioid epidemic. They were not sporadic or one-off stories. Each outlet devoted lots of attention to the opioid epidemic during the time span of 2015 to 2020. This span of time covers the third wave of the epidemic and the deadliest year of 2017. This also offers a bit of variety and different types of media to consider how the pain debate is being framed and reported on to the public. *Time* utilizes visuals and *NPR's All Things Considered* utilizes audio and visuals. I explore how those visuals impact the frames as well. The following chapter presents a brief sample of those articles. I will also offer a bit of background of the opioid epidemic with regard to prescribing practices that are at the heart of the pain management debate. I do not venture too deeply into the context of the opioid epidemic further than what the articles yield. There are amazing articles and books that cover the complex nature of how race and gender further complicate the epidemic. However, the articles included in this framing study do not discuss those dynamics, so I did not document them here.

THE OPIOID EPIDEMIC: A STORY OF PATIENTS, PRESCRIBERS, AND UNDERSTANDING PAIN IN AMERICA

Pain in America has been understood in different ways over the centuries. Before the 1990s, pain was not always viewed in America as a medical concern or even physical measure of health. For many people with pain, you just dealt with it at home and did not seek out a physician for treatment. Studies and new advocacy groups, such as the American Pain Society, began pushing for pharmacological remedies for pain in the average patient to become part of regular patient care in the early 1990s. Before then, pharmacological responses to pain were generally reserved for either cancer and terminally ill patients due to their addictive qualities and risks of side effects. According to Stephen A. Bernard et al., this shift marks the transition that lead to how the opioid epidemic became an epidemic:

> By the 1990s, the American Pain Society and other groups began developing guidelines for management of both acute and chronic pain that used mainly pharmaceutical approaches. Many of these groups (including the American Pain Society) received funding from Purdue Pharma, the manufacturer of Percodan (oxycodone and aspirin) and subsequently Oxycontin (long-acting oxycodone).[6]

This marked shift in prescribing practices is directly responsible for the epidemic. Access to the powerful drugs, patients thinking they were simply following doctor's orders, and doctors being misled about the addictive qualities of the prescribing all factor in in major ways. To assuage fears of prescribing, Bernard et al. found, "Purdue Pharma's representatives claimed that only 1 in 10,000 opioid-treated patients would become addicted if treated by a physician; no scientific data to support this was presented. Ultimately, Congressional hearings on the current opioid epidemic brought out information that Purdue Pharma knowingly disseminated false information."[7] Prescriptions for opioids rose steadily over the 1990s and then "quadrupled between 1999 and 2010, coinciding with a quadrupling in prescription-opioid-related deaths."[8]

Regarding the opioid epidemic, many people become addicted as a course of following their doctor's orders and taking a prescribed pain killer. Dr. Anna Lembke remarks, "For increasing numbers of people, especially young people, prescription drugs are the first exposure to addictive substances and the first stepping-stone to future addictive use."[9] Over 80 percent of heroin users were prescribed prescription opioid painkillers before they used heroin.[10] Furthermore, Dr. Lembke explains an underlying cause of the opioid epidemic. "The prescription drug epidemic is first and foremost an epidemic of overprescribing."[11] Nicholas D. Kristof and Sheryl WuDunn point to big pharma and prescribers receiving fiscal incentives to prescribe to drive the epidemic. Many doctors were unknowingly overprescribing due to erroneous reports and misleading information about the risks associated with pain killers.

The story of the opioid epidemic cannot be told without understanding the relationship between pharmaceutical companies and prescribers. Aggressive marketing, research endorsed by the very companies marketing these opioid pain killers, and incentives for doctors to prescribe particular brands drove the epidemic to its current state. With very little regulation of how or how much to prescribe, doctors were fueling the fire. Kristof and WuDunn explain:

> The story of America's current addiction nightmare begins in the 1990s, when the pharmaceutical industry was looking for a new blockbuster drug to market. . . . So, the pharmaceutical industry, led by Purdue Pharma and the Sackler family who owned it, marshaled a sophisticated campaign to treat pain more aggressively—with their opioid prescription pain killers.[12]

Before the 1990s, opioids for pain were mostly prescribed as palliative or hospice care at the end of life. This major shift in how pain was treated and understood culturally in America starting in the early 1990s and spiraled out of control by the dawning of the twenty-first century. Corporate greed made a new drug and simultaneously crafted a new market of unsuspecting patients and duped doctors. The pain debate often places culpability on pharmaceutical companies, but their voices can and do appear in the debate. In spite of the staggering evidence that these major corporations deceived doctors and created marketing materials that hid the dangers from patients, they fight in the debate as though there is something to be salvaged.

The marketing campaigns changed that perspective entirely and created a new market of patients through their novel drugs. Quite a market they created as well. As of 2014, "more than ten million Americans report non-medical use of prescription opiates and two million non-medical users of opiates meet criteria for substance use disorders."[13] As of 2019, Purdue Pharma is bankrupt after numerous lawsuits from states and individuals who suffered enormously from the erroneous and negligent marketing and incentives offered to doctors for prescribing these drugs. Kristoff and WuDunn argue, "Pharmaceutical companies commissioned reports arguing that doctors were allowing patient to suffer unnecessarily. There was an element of truth to this critique, and that recognition helped the pharmaceutical marketing campaign gain traction."[14] This indemnifies pain as suffering, rather than just a part of daily life in America, which it was widely viewed as for centuries by numerous Americans, particularly if a profession demanded physical labor. Aches and pain were considered par for the course and not a medical concern. Doctors take an oath to do no harm and the pharmaceutical companies were targeting that sentiment in their marketing techniques. The salience of pain as the new marker for evidence-based medicine and proper course of treatment including pain killers came from the producers of the pills themselves.

MEDIA FRAMING THEORY

How various media outlets are framing the pain debate is key for how the public will understand it. Robert Entman summarizes framing theory here:

> To frame is to *select some aspects of a perceived reality and make them more salient in a communicating text, in such a way as to promote a particular problem definition, causal interpretation, moral evaluation, and/or treatment recommendation* for the item described. Typically frames diagnose, evaluate, and prescribe.[15]

Framing narrows the perspective of complex issues. This is typical of most forms of media, but for reporting on an issue, can prove necessary for generating interesting articles while still informing the reader and/or listener. As they are notable trends in the rhetoric of in the other chapters, I used medicalization and legal as the frames to look for in articles. Search terms to include articles and ultimately determine the samples for the chapter were: chronic pain debate, doctor, patient, illicit, drug dealer, and pharmaceutical company. Each of these terms were notable and consistent in the other case studies in the other chapters with the exception of the chronic pain debate. I focused on these stories in particular to include in the chapter because they were the longest, to give more to work with for analysis, and had the tightest focus upon the chronic pain debate in the United States. The stories from *The New York Times, Time* magazine, and *NPR's All Things Considered* that appear in this chapter each were the longest of the articles my search yielded using *Lexis-Nexis* and had substantial usage of the terms for selection.

The diagnosing and prescribing portions of media framing theory are rather fitting for media that focuses on prescribers and patients for framing the debate about pain in the United States. The following analysis shows how the focus on the debate tends to stick to the two sides of siding with patients' access and rights or the scourge of addiction driving the public health emergency that is the opioid epidemic. Furthermore, stories about the pain debate frame prescribers and patients as the key players, relegating pharmaceutical companies to the background, though still framed as vital to the epidemic. Stories about the pain debate always feature a synecdoche of a patient suffering from chronic pain and a prescriber put at odds with the patient through new regulations and policies stemming from the opioid epidemic.

A BRIEF SAMPLE OF THE PAIN DEBATE PLAYED OUT IN THE MEDIA

Why America Can't Kick Its Painkiller Problem

Visuals and text matter to media framing immensely. This first example demonstrates the ways in which visuals can assist in the framing of the debate, enhance the medicalization narrative, and build compassion for the patient side of the debate significantly. The patient as synecdoche is a potent driver in the debate overall. This 2015 story in *Time* magazine, titled "Why America Can't Kick Its Painkiller Problem," demonstrates all of the key qualities of framing the pain debate. Because it is a magazine known for its images, a piece out of *Time* is a fitting place to start. First, after the title page, the audience sees a photograph of a woman looking out her living room window. The room is dimly lit and the woman looks depressed. The caption reads: "From patient to addict—When her doctor cut off her pain medication two years after a car accident, Tiffany Turner turned to the black market."[16] The visual and the textual message already has pitted patient rights to access against the prescriber. It implies blame to the doctor for denying access, which forced the patient to turn to the "black market," and pushed her into a more stigmatized drug addiction.

Tiffany Turner serves as a synecdoche for the opioid epidemic as well as the pain management debate. Her narrative is also medicalized in the *Time* article. The sentence, "from patient to addict," tells her medicalized narrative and primes the reader to be sympathetic. Tiffany's pain is not her fault and her lack of treatment is what forced her narrative arc to transition from a safe doctor's office to the world of illicit and dangerous street drugs. Because of the epidemic, Tiffany's pain has been ignored by doctors and broad strokes of a policy that underserves Tiffany, and patients like her. The reader can extrapolate out from Tiffany, the synecdoche, and imagine the many more people suffering from chronic pain who will be underserved and forced to turn to the black market and illicit drug addiction.

The two sides of the debate are already apparent in this story in *Time*. This particular article seems to choose the side of the patients, or at least expresses more sympathy for the patients' rights and access side. The medicalization narrative is strongly on the side of patients' rights to access medical solutions, including the opioid painkillers needed, and frames the public health policies meant to stymie the epidemic as part of the problem that leads to addiction to illicit drugs. The text continues on the following page:

> This is not a story about dark alleys and drug dealers. It starts in doctors' offices with everyday people seeking relief from pain and suffering. Around the nation,

> doctors so frequently prescribe the drugs known as opioids for chronic pain from conditions like arthritis, migraines and lower-back injuries that there are enough pills prescribed every year to keep every American adult medicated around the clock for a month.[17]

The path to addiction is telling and does not portray the patients involved in a negative light. It is not a moral failing, it is a medically framed issue, that starts with a medical problem and a legal prescription. The legal frame does come into the picture the article paints when they get to discussing the role of doctors in the opioid epidemic being largely due to their being duped by pharmaceutical companies:

> In some cases, regulators, doctors and patients were criminally misled into believing opioids were safe and effective. In 2007 the Department of Justice accused Purdue of deceptively telling doctors OxyContin was safer and less addictive than other drugs. The company and several executives pleaded guilty to misleading doctors and were fined $635 million.[18]

While important to include the history of the role of pharmaceutical companies and the legal ramifications of their marketing ploys, the reader would have to be rather invested and make it a few pages in before getting to this information in the article. The priming of the early framing that pits doctors against patients is more salient because of the arrangement of information and order of experiencing the information. Images in connection to text, such as the full-page image of Tiffany Turner and the caption, drive the attachment to memory of the consumer. In sum, the portion of the article with images and captions are the portions most likely to stay in the mind of the consumer after reading because of the power of images to impart an emotional connection.

Visuals play a strong role in influencing emotions. The medicalized narrative is supplemented by visuals in order to drive the synecdochal connection further. Instead of imagining, the *Time* article illustrates a rich picture of a sympathetic situation that many find themselves in. Tiffany's image becomes a visual synecdoche as well through the images shown. Barbie Zelizer explains this connection and interdependence of images, emotional connection, and words here, "dependence on words is enhanced and magnified in memory, where words provide order and connection."[19] The image and emotional stain from it sticks in the memory of the reader. Emma Frances Bloomfield and Angeline Sangalang cite, "the visual functions as an enthymeme that incorporates the audience in argument construction and as synecdoche that argues for the generalizability of images."[20] The caption categorizes and orders the connection the reader will have logged in their memory and enhances the power of the synecdoche of Tiffany's plight. So, the impact of that initial image and caption being the first thing the reader experiences is important to the framing of the pain debate as a whole. It centers the medicalization of a patient narrative and leaves an indelible impression.

Letter to the Editor RE "Taxpayer-Funded Addiction"

November 20, 2017, *The New York Times* ran a *Letter to the Editor* piece that illustrates some of the points of the pain debate from the reader's perspective. This series of articles is where the pharmaceutical representative makes themselves known and is present in the debate. Those who wrote in made sure to identify themselves and other relevant information to their response to an earlier article. Stephen J. Ubl from Washington starts off the article by stating "Effectively addressing the opioid crisis requires a comprehensive approach that meets immediate needs and invests in future solutions for patients."[21] Right in the first line, the side of the debate is clearly expressed. Ubl then moves to explain that "the biopharmaceutical industry can and should play a unique role. Our industry is developing 40 nonopioid analgesics and has an additional 40 addiction recovery treatments in the pipeline. The National Institutes of Health and the National Institute on Drug Abuse are wrestling with this problem as well, and working in partnership we can solve it."[22] The writer's byline becomes even more relevant at this juncture of reading his portion of the article. Ubl is president and chief executive of Pharmaceutical Research and Manufacturers of America. Though the industry is in part culpable, that fades into the background so much so that it is nonexistent in this response, and it is argued that the pharmaceutical companies be a part of the solution. This certainly follows the medical framing and sides with the patient's rights and access side of the debate. The argument is that pharmaceutical companies can and are producing new drugs that nonopioids and still treat pain.

The next writer in this piece is also, wait for it, from the pharmaceutical industry. It is interesting to see them use this as free advertising for their cause. *The New York Times* is quite the platform as well. This writer's piece takes a slightly different tack than the first. Craig Landau, an anesthesiologist, president, and chief executive of Purdue Pharma, defends his industry. Here Landau proclaims his detest, "We disagree with the opinion expressed by a pharmacologist in the editorial that 'abuse-deterrent is a marketing term used to mislead.' 'Opioid medicines with abuse-deterrent properties' is a designation by the Food and Drug Administration, described in the final 'Guidance for Industry' for products having specific properties designed to deter their abuse by certain routes."[23] He also, before defending his industry, demands that patients' rights and access to medication to treat pain by stating, "We must address this crisis without abandoning pain patients."[24] The side of the debate is immediately recognizable and the perspective of defense of the pharmaceutical companies is a bit of an outlier in comparison to the others.

The patient synecdoche is present in *the New York Times* article as well. The side of patients' rights in the next portion of the article comes directly from a patient herself. Suzanne Fessenden concludes her letter by stating, "Doctors, do your jobs, follow guidelines, but keep in mind that not all patients are drug seekers; some are using the drug as it was developed to be used and are grateful for its existence."[25] The testimony of a patient is powerful here. Suzanne is calling out doctors in particular and even thanks her own physician who, "despite pressures to decrease oxycodone prescriptions recognizes that not all patients are addicts."[26] This portion breaks from the medical frame and places responsibility on doctors as well as patients to be "good" patients who follow instructions as she has. This stands out in stark contrast from the presentation in the *Time* article. The *Time* article suggests that even while following directions, the dangerous class of drugs that opioids are presents the issue, and makes clear that it is not a "drug seeker" behavior, but a consequence of opioid use in general. Suzanne stands in as the synecdoche of the responsible patient, not the drug seeker, who is ruining it for the responsible ones. The medicalized narrative is prominent here and emphasizes that patients are still patients, doctors should follow guidelines, but should also know how to tell a difference in their *good* and their *bad* patients. This exemplifies the hold-overs from prior policies that are punitive and reflects that sentiments about drug use are still highly stigmatized in America.

The final section is the only nonpharmaceutically linked doctor's opinion. Steven A. King, a pain management physician, begins his letter on the side of doctors in the debate. King's letter concludes by offering rationale for how a doctor may misunderstand or be gullible to marketing ploys from pharmaceutical companies, "Most physicians receive little education and training in pain management in medical school and postgraduate training."[27] King points to nonopioid pain management that is often "far more effective than opioids" as directions that doctors should take and patients should ask for.[28] According to King, there are many alternatives to opioids that could assist with pain management and are safer, nonaddictive paths to upholding patients' rights and getting around the issue of opioids.

Opioids Don't Beat Other Medications for Chronic Pain

On a March 6, 2018 broadcast from the *National Public Radio's* series *All Things Considered,* host Mary Louise Kelly begins the show by telling listeners about a new study: "OK, from the toll of opioid addiction to pain relief. In the minds of many people, these drugs remain the champions for relieving the worst pain. But a new study shows that when it comes to chronic pain, opioids actually work no better than nonopioid drugs."[29] The opening line of the broadcast suggests a perspective on the debate that is on the side of looking at the impacts of the opioid epidemic and finding alternative solutions to chronic pain. The third line down in the transcript shows testimony from a chronic pain sufferer named Renea Molden. Her doctor took her off of opioid pills and her immediate reaction was anger: "I was mad. I'll be honest. I was mad. I was frustrated." This shift immediately into the account of a patient's perspective shifts the perspective to the side of the debate that is for patients' rights and access. But the pendulum swings again to reveal a new study that demonstrates that nonopioid pain treatments are actually more effective and have fewer side effects. The balance continues throughout the episode. Which is fairly typical of the *All Things Considered* series.

The doctor running the study, Dr. Erin Krebs, is interviewed and her voice is present in the series. Dr. Krebs breaks the message down simply here, "The bottom line in terms of the message for people who have chronic back pain or arthritis pain is just that you shouldn't start opioids. For most people, they just have extra risk and no extra benefit compared with nonopioid medications."[30] By 2018, more and more studies regarding the efficacy of opioids, not coming from pharmaceutical companies, were on the rise. The demand that the opioid epidemic and public health emergency put on the country elevated the need for these types of studies. Balancing patients' rights and access to pain management while stymying the tide of the epidemic seem to be getting more balanced, but there is still a long road of transitioning patients to nonopioid medications.

Another doctor, Dr. Muhammad Farhan of Kansas City, is featured in an interview. Dr. Farhan is the head of a pain clinic and does not use opioids. Alternative approaches, such as mindfulness and meditation, as well as nonopioid medications are all that is used. Dr. Farhan reports, "Most of the time what I see is that they are taking high doses of opioids. Then they're in bed all the time or sleeping and still in pain."[31] Even without the pressures of the opioid epidemic, it seems like these patients would still be there, needing relief that opioids did not provide. This is another perspective of a patient's access to pain treatment who did not see success and relief, like Renea Molden did, and still the field of medicine needs to advance to give them higher quality of life. The medical framing is clearly in place and the value of our society to live a life free of pain is also present.

Overall, this representative anecdote of a complex and sprawling debate offers a picture of how the debate is going. The representation of perspectives in the pain management debate in the United States reveals much about how the medicalization narrative can take a slightly different turn. The debate often is framed in a way that puts doctors and patients at odds with one another. Policies, new laws, and programs to curtail prescribing opioids in general are framed as a medical issue, a public health issue, and a patients' rights issue. The *Letter to the Editor* article in *The New York Times* had actual representatives from the pharmaceutical industry defending their approaches to marketing opioids. In the *Time* piece and the *All Things Considered* broadcast, pharmaceutical companies were not framed favorably and blame is placed upon them for their greed and misleading marketing tactics that duped doctors across the country. By 2011, the overprescribing issue had become rampant. Dr. Anna Lembke remarks of the alarming rate of prescribing opioid painkillers by doctors as well as the climbing death rate associated with their use:

> the Centers for Disease Control (CDC), the agency of the government responsible for protecting Americans from major health threats, declared a "prescription drug epidemic"; and the CDC was unequivocal about what had caused this epidemic: "prescription opioid painkillers and psychotherapeutic drugs being prescribed more widely by physicians." In the United States, approximately 4,000 deaths involving opioid painkillers were documented in 1999, increasing to 16, 235 in 2013, quadrupling in little more than a decade.[32]

The location of blame upon pharmaceutical companies and doctors is understandable. It bears out in the statistics and governmental agency findings consistently.

The *Time* article used a legal frame and pointed to the criminality and deception they were found guilty of in courts of law. The *All Things Considered* broadcast featured very little information about pharmaceutical companies, but concluded that there are more effective pain management therapies available that do not include opioids. In fact, opioids are not effective for pain management and are just dangerous. Doctors also were allowed within the sympathetic medicalization narrative as experts in the search for alternatives to opioid painkillers and allies of pain patients. The patients and doctors were on the same side of the debate in the *All Things Considered* piece. The interviews demonstrate that both had been left to find new pathways after the pharmaceutical companies' deceptions and the new legislation that limited access to dangerous opioid painkillers. One thread ran through all of the stories: each contained a medicalized narrative that framed pain as something that no one should have to experience. That cultural and societal value was not questioned.

PAIN IN AMERICA

The rhetorical treatment of the opioid epidemic in these news stories is rather revealing when it comes to understanding our cultural and societal views of pain in America. Pain seems to be an important lynchpin in how the epidemic got to where it is currently. Pain is a real struggle for millions of Americans. The medical profession seemed woefully unprepared for the cultural shifts that brought pain patients to them. The pharmaceutical companies with deceptive practices seemed more than willing to meet the demand and even craft it through flawed research and outright deceptive marketing strategies. Pain leads to feelings of isolation, loss of worth, loss of a sense of self, and a whole host of psychological maladies such as depression and anxiety. Zoorob and Salemi offer a hopeful suggestion to stave off substance use disorder rates and the seeking of pain drugs to start with. Their research found that "low social capital" underlay both seeking out prescription painkillers and misuse of those. Their study expands understanding pain and isolation as motivators for seeking out opioid painkillers in the first place:

> by suggesting that social capital promotes community resilience. This research can inform policymaking towards the opiate epidemic in two ways. First, since social capital may mollify drug epidemics, policymakers would be well-advised to consider how to facilitate its growth. Second, communities with little social capital are particularly vulnerable to drug epidemics, and treatment and prevention efforts should be targeted accordingly.[33]

Pain clearly leads people to seek out chemical solutions. Perhaps steps to shore up the declining social capital in America is a solution that the pain debate is missing.

Something has to give in the fight against the opioid epidemic. The pain management debate reveals interesting framing that limits our view of the issue at hand. Cutting off the supply of opioid pain killers and finding new, innovative ways to treat pain are both valid. Medicalization narratives and patient synecdoche are certainly effective approaches and merited in the debate. But what about the underlying social and cultural frames that got us to the point of an epidemic in the first place? I propose that we as a society reevaluate our framing of pain and are critical of the frames used. Perhaps, if we reframe and refocus our attention on new ways to frame the issue, we can discover new ways to cope with pain and suffering in order to develop a healthier society overall.

NOTES

1. *One Nation Under Stress: Deaths of Despair in the United States*, directed by Marc Levin and Daphne Pinkerson (New York City, NY: HBO Documentary Films, 2019), Streaming.

2. German Lopez, "The Debate over Prescription Painkillers, Explained," *Vox*, July 5, 2015, https://www.vox.com/2015/5/15/8611703/the-debate-over-prescription-painkillers-explained.

3. Andrew Rosenblum, Lisa A. March, Herman Joseph, and Russell K. Portenoy, "Opioids and the Treatment of Chronic Pain: Controversies, Current Status, and Future Directions," *Expert Clinical Psychopharmacology* 16 (5), (2008): 409.

4. Ibid, 407.

5. "Data Overview: Overview of the Drug Overdose Epidemic: Behind the Numbers," Opioid Overdose, Centers for Disease Control and Prevention, 2019, https://www.cdc.gov/drugoverdose/data/index.html.

6. Stephen A. Bernard, Paul R. Chelminski, Timothy J. Ives, and Shabbar I. Ranapurwala, "Management of Pain in the United States—A Brief History and Implications for the Opioid Epidemic," *Health Services Insights* 11, (2018): 2.

7. Ibid, 4.

8. Anna Lembke, *Drug Dealer, MD* (Baltimore: Johns Hopkins University Press, 2016), 4.

9. Ibid, 23.

10. Stephen A. Bernard, Paul R. Chelminski, Timothy J. Ives, and Shabbar I. Ranapurwala, "Management of Pain in the United States—A Brief History and Implications for the Opioid Epidemic," *Health Services Insights* 11 (2018): 6.

11. Ibid, 25.

12. Nicholas D. Kristof and Sheryl WuDunn, *Tightrope: Americans Reaching for Hope* (New York: Alfred A. Knopf, 2020), 80.

13. Michael J. Zoorob and Jason L. Salemi, "Bowling Alone, Dying Together: The Role of Social Capital in Mitigating the Drug Overdose Epidemic in the United States," *Drug and Alcohol Dependence* 173, (2017): 1.

14. Ibid, 80.

15. Robert M. Entman, "Framing: Toward Clarification of a Fractured Paradigm," *Journal of Communication* 43 (4), (1993): 52.

16. Massimo Calabresi, "Why America Can't Kick Its Painkiller Problem." *Time*, June 15, 2015, 27.

17. Ibid, 28.

18. Ibid, 31.

19. Barbie Zelizer, *Remembering to Forget: Holocaust Memory Through the Camera's Eye* (Chicago: The University of Chicago Press, 1998), 5.

20. Emma Frances Bloomfield and Angeline Sangalang, "Juxtaposition as Visual Argument: Health Rhetoric in Super Size Me and Fat Head," *Argumentation & Advocacy* 50 (3), (2014): 142.

21. "Pain Management and the Opioid Crisis." *New York Times*, November 20, 2017, A22(L).

22. Ibid.
23. Ibid.
24. Ibid.
25. Ibid.
26. Ibid.
27. Ibid.
28. Ibid.
29. "Opioids Don't Beat Other Medications For Chronic Pain." *All Things Considered*, March 6, 2018.
30. Ibid.
31. Ibid.
32. Anna Lembke, *Drug Dealer, MD* (Baltimore: Johns Hopkins University Press, 2016), 4.
33. Michael J. Zoorob and Jason L. Salemi, "Bowling Alone, Dying Together: The Role of Social Capital in Mitigating the Drug Overdose Epidemic in the United States," *Drug and Alcohol Dependence* 173 (2017): 8.

Conclusion

A Very American Epidemic

Rhetoric of the Opioid Epidemic

The interconnected case studies represent the broader ways in which the rhetoric of the opioid epidemic is articulated in this moment in time. The public health frame and medicalization of the issue of opioid use in America is rather revealing. There is a strong presence of synecdoches that reinforce medicalization narratives, public health framing, and assert that the epidemic *is* indeed an epidemic, not a drug issue. These representations can move us rhetorically as a society and culture in a productive manner away from the old, ineffective rhetoric of the "war on drugs." We as a society can demand our government, law enforcement, and public health officials deal with the opioid epidemic accordingly. But there is still much work to be done to shift the cultural and societal understandings in America of the epidemic.

Unlike approaches to and early representations of the rampant issue and devastations of crack cocaine use in the 1980s, recent devastations associated with opioid use have benefited from public health frames and fairly early medicalization of the problem. Rather than criminality frames being dominant, the opioid epidemic has been treated as that: an epidemic. This is due to a large contributing factor to the epidemic being overprescribing by medical doctors and patients unwittingly becoming addicted to opioids while following a doctor's orders. Once addicted and when the supply of prescribed opioids dried up, patients then often turned to other methods of procuring opioids and often turned to other modalities of opioids. According to Finkelman and McGinnis:

> as the supply of prescription opioids was curtailed, prices of the drugs rose and overall access became more difficult. In turn, those who had become addicted to prescription opioids turned to cheaper, more accessible, and more potent drugs, such as heroin. Between 2003 and 2013, an estimated three out of four new heroin users reported previous misuse of prescription opioids prior to using heroin.[1]

Another is that non-Hispanic white Americans were the first predominant group cited as having the most significant change in outcomes of health and morbidity. That rhetorically demands particular approaches that tend to be more medically-oriented, are derived from public health, work against stigma associated with drug use and addiction treatment, and contain more compassion than seen in the United States in previous decades.

The governmental and news media representation of the pain debates is not as consistent as the popular culture case studies. This is particularly troubling thinking through the way funding is sourced from the highest level of government down. The Trump administration promised to add funds and end the epidemic, but the epidemic raged on. Trump's rhetoric reflected the out of date and ineffective legal and criminality frames from the war on drugs. Even with a drug epidemic that, at the time of Trump delivering the speech, effected more non-Hispanic whites than any other demographic, the criminality and legal frames held steady. Fearing the criminal other morphed into fearing the criminal other that holds a prescription pad. Indicting medical doctors and holding them side by side to drug dealers was a main point from Trump's speech. This holds rhetorical potential to undercut the medical approach completely that he lauds by way of dispensing Narcan, an overdose reversal medication, and putting trust into pharmaceutical companies to make an *actually* nonaddictive pain medication this time. Trump's rhetorical approach forgets the pharmaceutical companies' roles in touting opioid pain killers as nonaddictive and muddies any hope of a clear message about how to stop the opioid epidemic.

In contrast, the popular culture case studies consistently use medicalization narratives and the public health framing is firm. The powerful synecdoches featured in both the documentaries and *Ben is Back* support the medicalization and public health frames in productive ways. The epidemic, according to these case studies, *is* a public health issue and one that ought to be approached medically, behaviorally, and through mental health support. The underlying causes are diverse and complex in these popular media representative anecdotes. In part because each of those examples looks at the placement of blame in pharmaceutical company greed, the misleading information and incentives presented to doctors, and patients looking for solutions to their despair and pain. The rhetoric of medicalization and public health framing presents the field of medicine as simultaneously a cause and a solution. The films, however, do not shy away from presenting that complexity and use it as a way to point out the flaws in our current healthcare system in the United States. How to progress medicine in ways that address despair, pain, and addiction more productively were areas highlighted. Furthermore, stigma was addressed head on and efforts were made to reduce it through the powerful synecdoches that were easy to identify with were consistent. On the other hand, the governmental representations were inconsistent and mixed. The news media representation of the pain debate also adds to stigma of addiction in ways that may muddle the public health framing and medicalization narratives. Presenting the issue of chronic pain in this manner can bring to bear a confusion about whether or not the medical field is even prepared to be a solution. Solutions were offered in the presentation of the debate, but were not the focus of the stories. Rather, focusing on the narrative of victims of either side of the debate took focus. At least focusing upon individual narratives as representative anecdotes produces a humanizing rhetoric and does not flatten them into "addicts" writ large.

Discursive productions of the issue as an *epidemic* works to persuasively channel perceptions, direct policy decisions, shape approaches to solving the epidemic, and ultimately impact broader cultural, political, and economic understandings of opioid use overall. The opioid epidemic as a symptom of our how our nation operates is a telling one. Understanding the underlying causes of the opioid epidemic and how to remedy them will, I believe, make us stronger as a nation if we can address them productively and with compassion.

SUMMARY OF ANALYSIS FINDINGS

The most intriguing, as far as revealing that we still have a long way to go rhetorically as well as literally in our approach to resolve the epidemic, was Trump's speech *Remarks on Combating the Opioid Crisis*. The tenuous ways in which our President rhetorically handles the epidemic is highly problematic and reinforces stigma about the issue. By locating solutions such as the death penalty, traditional law enforcement strategies borrowed from prior drug issues in America, and the securitization framing to the opioid crisis, this ultimately digresses the issue. While it is important to stop the supply of deadly substances into the United States, the focal point and framing of the issue through solutions based in old, "war on drugs" approaches—that have been largely substantiated as ineffective—do not assist with ending the epidemic. Though the victims of the crisis, that filled very little time in the speech, are not blamed, the focus on solutions that are punitive stick with old, problematic frames. The public health frame and medicalization narratives were represented the least in this case study. It is still a productive rhetorical analysis to demonstrate how there are slippages in the approach to the epidemic. Even the President calls the epidemic a crisis more in the speech, in spite of declaring it a public health emergency. The framing of the matter in the speech rhetorically undermines the declaration of his own administration.

Novel approaches that adapt law enforcement, first responders, and government officials' roles to adequately address the opioid epidemic came through strongly in the case study of ODMAP. Created by HIDTA in Washington D.C., the ODMAP technology adapts the role and approaches of law enforcement to be that of a progressive public health approach. Punitive approaches are dropped in favor of medical ones. ODMAP assists with tracking the flow of drugs and spikes in deadly drug use, certainly, but it does so in the pursuit of connecting sufferers with medical, behavioral, and mental health supports they need to fully recover. Naloxone is front and center of the map and assists with providing more supplies of Naloxone to the areas of the country that need it most. The mapping technology also mirrors traditional disease tracking maps and technology that assist with tracking, containing, and ending epidemics. The public health frame and medicalization are firmly strategies that are visually, textually, and verbally reinforced at every juncture of the map and the website that supports law enforcement, first responders, and public health officials to implement it. The epideictic and communal functions of the map are rather intriguing as it builds a coalition of individual agencies whom wish to implement progressive policy to end the epidemic. The map demonstrates the bond of these agencies through a shared goal: medically moving the epidemic to a stopping point and saving lives.

The pain debate is squarely framed as medical with strong public health approaches as the focal point. The media coverage of the pain debate demonstrates that there are strong opinions about the shifts in medicine that the opioid epidemic has brought about and public health approaches. It serves as a synecdoche for how patients, doctors, pharmaceutical companies, and stigma clash as we work through how to end the epidemic. While the public health approach and medical nature of the epidemic are not questioned, this case study brought up some important cultural and societal facets of the epidemic. Patients, for example, are not all rhetorically treated the same. Patients' medicalized narratives serve as productive synecdoches for the opioid epidemic, but there are some tenuous spots where patients' medicalized narratives are split into categories—the "good" patient and the "drug seeking" patient—that reveal that there is still a long ways to go to undo the stigma of drug use in America.

Popular media sources are key for spreading information and persuading the nation about how to view the opioid epidemic. Bloomfield and Sangalang assert, "Health issues are also being addressed in the realm of entertainment. Documentary films in particular (i.e., *Food, Inc., Killer at Large,* and *Food Fight)* are an accessible source of health information for the public (Nisbet & Aufderheide, 2009)."[2] The popular media representations were also consistent in the framing of the opioid epidemic as a medical issue that demands a public health approach, compassion, and progressive policy to end it. Each popular representation also actively recognized the stigmas of drug use in America and address it by breaking it down and *representing it as a medical issue, not a criminal one. One Nation Under Stress* and *Heroin(e)* are both firmly fighting against misunderstandings and poor perceptions about opioid use in America. The synecdochal arguments in each are compelling and serve as productive representative anecdotes to assist in understanding the opioid epidemic in a way that is not overwhelming.

Each documentary explores the complex dynamics of underlying causes in a way that is accessible. Both highlight the role of pharmaceutical companies, doctor's prescribing processes, and the ways in which society and the government has underserved the demographics hardest hit by the epidemic. *Heroin(e)* leans on synecdoche by virtue of focusing on one of the hardest hit areas in the nation, West Virginia, and by featuring medicalization narratives. *One Nation Under Stress* emphasizes the medical underpinnings of how we understand pain in America and the confluence of this understanding and the greed of pharmaceutical companies allowed to mislead and market deadly, addictive substances with little to no oversight. In each documentary, experts guide the audience to a better understanding of what the opioid epidemic is and how a compassionate, medicalized, public health-centric approach is the only way to stymie the tide of opioid use and death. These experts are also the very ones rhetorically charged and demonstrated to be effective in the way out of the epidemic: a medical doctor and first responder. By having these experts be the main people the audience is invited to identify with, the audience takes on their perspective and that of the medicalization and public health framing of the epidemic.

There are only a handful of popular films and series that tackle the opioid epidemic. *Ben is Back* is a synecdoche for the epidemic that operates rhetorically to dispense information about the epidemic in a dramatic, emotionally-charged, entertaining way. It also is persuading viewers to view and feel about the epidemic in very particular ways. Holly, the mother of a sufferer of opioid use disorder, is the main character the audience identifies with. Her experience and approach to the epidemic that her son is stuck in the grips of is how we, the viewer, thereby experience the epidemic through this medium. The medicalization narrative and public health frame is firmly in place throughout the film and reinforced in key scenes that are emotionally powerful. Using a star-studded cast of actors, such as Julia Roberts and Lucas Hedges, in a family drama from a director well-known for them guarantees an audience. The synecdoche of Holly's personal and family's experience with the epidemic makes it relatable and approachable. This allows for the public health framing and medicalized narrative to even be welcomed by those whom may have misperceptions and negative feelings about the epidemic.

LESSONS LEARNED

As a rhetoric and media scholar, I was fascinated when my partner came home and told me about his days at work dealing with the epidemic head on as someone in the public health field. Through a state funded grant, he was put in charge of developing and implementing a plan to get Narcan—a brand name for the Naloxone overdose reversal medication mentioned numerous times in the analysis chapters—out to those who needed it in Marion County. He then explained to me some of his newly acquired knowledge about *deaths of despair.* The curious researcher in me was immediately hooked. What a rhetorically charged way to put it: deaths of despair. Also, how bleak and depressing. I needed to know more.

I realized as I got into the project how much I had already been exposed to deaths of despair. By the time I was in middle school I had already lost two peers to suicide. One was an overdose of pain pills and one was more violent and physically induced. I never learned which pills, but I was only thirteen at the time, and did not inquire further. The opioid portion of deaths of despair was already in my life at a young age. Philip Seymour Hoffman's sudden overdose death of heroin in 2014 years after being in recovery was a somber day. I remember the day Prince died as well. I was left wondering what fentanyl was and why it was put into pills that were labeled as other medications. Anthony Bourdain's suicide was a shock too. Chris Cornell's sudden death in 2017 was another one that shocked me. Vicky Cornell, his widow, blamed her husband's death on prescription pills. Vicky explains in an interview shortly after her husband's death, "Addiction is a disease."[3] This sentiment of the medicalization and public health framing of addiction is one of the main themes I found analyzing texts responding to the opioid epidemic. I also learned how steeped we are, no matter if we are directly experiencing the epidemic or not, it is everywhere in the United States and how varied perceptions of the epidemic can be.

I learned a lot while researching deaths of despair and analyzing various opioid epidemic texts. Most of all, I learned how fitting the term *deaths of despair* really is. Broad lessons are that the epidemic is referred to as an *epidemic* because so many of the underlying causes are firmly rooted in medical contexts. The beginnings of the supply of opioids to so many patients is rooted in the medical field and formerly trusted institutions such as pharmaceutical companies and pharmacies. Dr. Anna Lembke, during an interview with *NPR Fresh Air*'s Terry Gross, says "Starting in the 1980s, doctors started to be told that opioids were effective treatment for chronic pain, and that treating patients long-term with opioids was evidence-based medicine. . . . That was patently false and that was propagated by what I call 'big medicine,' in cahoots with Big Pharma."[4] The beginnings of the epidemic clearly have a connection with overprescribing. Which means that plenty of those currently addicted to opioids were simply following doctor's orders and that doctors were following the information, or rather *propaganda* as Dr. Lembke describes it, from pharmaceutical companies. Case and Deaton cite pharmaceutical companies as one of the entities that has benefited in all of this, "We should note that a central beneficiary of opioids are the pharmaceutical companies that have promoted their sales. According to Harriet Ryan, Lisa Girion, and Scott Glover (2016), Purdue Pharmaceutical had earned $31 billion from sales of OxyContin as of mid-2016."[5] Corporate greed assisted in the United States' most costly epidemic to date, in terms of lives and economics. Before the COVID-19 pandemic was declared in March of 2020, the opioid epidemic was the largest public health issue in the United States.

Big pharma had also played a significant role in stymying efforts to control and limit the prescribing of opioids. Now that a few major companies have had to declare bankruptcy, the reckoning is here. Their role in perpetuating the issue is, hopefully, concluded. In spite of this shift, chapter 3 reveals that voices of chief executives from the pharmaceutical were present. Guised as sympathetic advocates arguing for the rights of patients, they are still finding outlets for defending pharmaceutical company marketing tactics as merely informative. Before writing this book, I was completely unaware that there was a debate over chronic pain management. As someone who suffers from chronic pain, I thought I would have heard something about it. Writer for *The New York Times,* Barry Meier, reports on multiple new bills and legislation moving swiftly in 2011 and 2012. So swiftly that it caught state legislatures off guard and ultimately thwarted the efforts pharmaceutical giants such as "The maker of OxyContin, Purdue Pharma, tried and failed to stop it. Several national pain experts, including some with ties to the drug industry, also sought to block it, saying the new provisions would cause chaos by restricting patient access to care."[6] It is important to note that the article specifies that it was doctors with ties to the drug industry making this complaint about patients being negatively impacted by the new prescribing laws, programs to limit the number of pills prescribed, and drug monitoring. Purdue Pharmaceuticals declared bankruptcy after a litany of legal suits lost. *CNN*'s Elizabeth Joseph reports, "Purdue Pharma, maker of the painkiller OxyContin, said its bankruptcy filing Sunday is part of an agreement to pay billions of dollars to states and local and tribal governments. The company has denied any wrongdoing."[7] Regardless of this development, the pain debate in the United States wages on.

Complications are many and there seem to be too many setbacks to articulate finding our way to the end of the opioid epidemic. Even worse, the opioid epidemic is being complicated further by the pandemic. The pandemic is not only causing a clear strain on the healthcare system charged with assisting those suffering from opioid use disorder, our society, economy, and nation as a whole is being set back significantly. A *National Geographic* article sums up the additional problems and implications for the opioid epidemic: "Amid widespread strains on the healthcare system, the United States remains in an overdose crisis—more than two million Americans use opioids . . . While COVID-19 has a disproportionate impact on various vulnerable populations, people with drug addictions are facing unique challenges in response to COVID-19."[8] The medical field is largely underprepared for one epidemic at a time, let alone a pandemic and epidemic happening concurrently, with the limited resources we as a society and government have allotted to adequate healthcare.

What stands out me to most is that the opioid epidemic is not a *drug* problem. It is much more of a societal and cultural problem. It is also a medical and public health issue, not one of incarceration and punitive approaches, but one that demands something much more nuanced and complex. Addiction to opioids seems to be more of a symptom than the cause of the epidemic. A symptom that reveals the nasty truth of life in the United States. Furthermore, it tells us something significant about life in America. The numerous inequities underlying the opioid epidemic cast doubt, for me at least, on the American dream. As someone who falls into the elder millennial age range as I write, I have felt the dashed expectations of the promises that have fell through, in spite of my pursuits of education and hard work. Case and Deaton sum up my sentiment in far more sophisticated language as they explain the unraveling of American society that began in the 1970s:

> Behind this lie familiar stories about globalization and automation, changes in social customs that have allowed dysfunctional changes in patterns of marriage and childrearing, the decline of unions, and others. Ultimately, we see our story as about the collapse of the white working class after its heyday in the early 1970s, and the pathologies that accompany this decline.[9]

Sadly, this epidemic does not have an end in sight. Some of Dr. Sanjay Gupta's concluding remarks in the documentary *One Nation Under Stress* resonate with me clearly. Dr. Gupta remarks, "We could stop manufacturing the disease in the first place."[10] That effort to stop manufacturing the disease—combined with the medical-behavioral approach and compassion found as themes throughout most of the texts analyzed—may be what it takes to find a solution to this very American opioid epidemic.

NOTES

1. Elizabeth M. Finkelman and J. Michael McGinnis, "The Emergence of an Epidemic." In *A Public Health Guide to Ending the Opioid Epidemic*, edited by Jay C. Butler, and Michael R. Fraser (Oxford: Oxford University Press, 2019), 13.

2. Emma Frances Bloomfield and Angeline Sangalang, "Juxtaposition as Visual Argument: Health Rhetoric in Super Size Me and Fat Head," *Argumentation & Advocacy* 50 (3), (2014): 141.

3. Daniel Kreps, "Chris Cornell's Widow Breaks Silence on Singer's Death, 'Addiction,'" *Rolling Stone,* June 28, 2017, https://www.rollingstone.com/music/music-news/chris-cornells-widow-breaks-silence-on-singers-death-addiction-201345/.

4. Terry Gross, "'Drug Dealer, M.D.': Misunderstandings and Good Intentions Fueled Opioid Epidemic," *Fresh Air-NPR,* December 15, 2016, https://www.npr.org/sections/health-shots/2016/12/15/505710073/drug-dealer-md-contends-that-well-meaning-docs-drove-the-opioid-epidemic.

5. Anne Case and Angus Deaton, "Mortality and Morbidity in the 21st Century," *Brookings Papers on Economic Activity*, Spring (2017): 433.

6. Barry Meier, "Tightening the Lid on Pain Prescriptions," *The New York Times,* April 8, 2012, https://alliance-primo.hosted.exlibrisgroup.com/permalink/f/e3ml1m/TN_gale_ofa285683281.

7. Elizabeth Joseph, "Purdue Pharma Files for Bankruptcy as Part of a $10 billion Agreement to Settle Opioid Lawsuits," *CNN,* September 16, 2019, https://www.cnn.com/2019/09/16/us/purdue-pharma-bankruptcy-filing/index.html.

8. Lois Parshley, "The Pandemic May Fuel the Next Wave of the Opioid Crisis," *National Geographic,* April 21, 2020, https://apple.news/AP1p3R64ES9So4tBOR-pdVA.

9. Anne Case and Angus Deaton, "Mortality and Morbidity in the 21st Century," *Brookings Papers on Economic Activity*, Spring (2017): 438–49.

10. *One Nation Under Stress: Deaths of Despair in the United States*, directed by Marc Levin and Daphne Pinkerson (New York City, NY: HBO Documentary Films, 2019), Streaming.

Bibliography

"5-Point Strategy to Combat the Opioid Crisis." *U.S. Department of Health and Human Services,* August 7, 2018, https://www.hhs.gov/opioids/about-the-epidemic/hhs-response/index.html.

Achenbach, Joel and Keating, Dan. "A New Divide in American Death." *The Washington Post*, April 10, 2016, online multimedia story, https://www.washingtonpost.com/sf/national/2016/04/10/a-new-divide-in-american-death/?utm_term=.6b948ce6c5e4.

Barney, Timothy. """'Gulag'—Slavery, Inc.": The Power of Place and the Rhetorical Life of a Cold War Map." *Rhetoric & Public Affairs* 16 (2), (2013): 321.

Bateman, John A. and Schmidt, Karl-Heinrich. *Multimodal Film Analysis How Films Mean* (New York: Routledge, 2012).

Beeson, Jeff. "ODMAP: A Digital Tool to Track and Analyze Overdoses." *National Institute of Justice,* May 14, 2018, https://nij.ojp.gov/topics/articles/odmap-digital-tool-track-and-analyze-overdoses.

Benson, Thomas. "The Rhetorical Structure of Frederick Wiseman's Primate." *The Quarterly Journal of Speech* 71 (2), (1985): 215.

Bernard, Stephen A., Paul R. Chelminski, Timothy J. Ives, and Shabbar I. Ranapurwala. "Management of Pain in the United States—A Brief History and Implications for the Opioid Epidemic." *Health Services Insights* 11 (2018): 1–6.

Blakemore, Erin. "Neuroscientists Think One Way to Fight Opioid Addiction is to Tackle Loneliness." *The Washington Post,* December 1, 2018. https://www.washingtonpost.com/national/health-science/neuroscientist-thinks-one-way-to-fight-opioid-addiction-is-to-tackle-loneliness/2018/11/30/8f651440-f33d-11e8-80d0-f7e1948d55f4_story.html.

Bloomfield, Emma Frances, and Angeline Sangalang. "Juxtaposition as Visual Argument: Health Rhetoric in Super Size Me and Fat Head." *Argumentation & Advocacy* 50 (3), (2014): 141–56.

Bostdorff, Denise M. "Epideictic Rhetoric in the Service of War: George W. Bush on Iraq and the 60th Anniversary of the Victory over Japan." *Communication Monographs* 78 (3), (2011): 297.

Botticelli, Michael, and Colleen L. Barry. "Stigma and the Language of Addiction." In *A Public Health Guide to Ending the Opioid Epidemic*, edited by Jay C. Butler, and Michael R. Fraser (Oxford University Press, 2019).

Burke, Kenneth. *A Grammar of Motives* (Berkeley: The University of California Press, 1969).

Burke, Kenneth. "Four Master Tropes." In *A Grammar of Motives* (Berkeley: University of California Press, 1945).

Butler, Jay C., and Michael R. Fraser. *A Public Health Guide to Ending the Opioid Epidemic* (New York, NY: Oxford University Press, 2019).

Calabresi, Massimo. "Why America Can't Kick Its Painkiller Problem." *Time*, June 15, 2015. Gale OneFile: Popular Magazines (accessed April 1, 2020).

Carr, Tom. "Fighting the Opioid Epidemic with ODMAP." *Washington/Baltimore High-Intensity Drug Trafficking Area,* Spring 2017, http://proceedings.esri.com/library/userconf/nss17/papers/nss_02.pdf.

Case, Anne and Angus Deaton. *Deaths of Despair and the Future of Capitalism* (New Jersey: Princeton University Press, 2020).

Case, Anne and Angus Deaton. "Mortality and Morbidity in the 21st Century." *Brookings Papers on Economic Activity* (Spring 2017): 399.

"Celebrating Lost Loved Ones." *esri,* 2019, https://opioidepidemic.maps.arcgis.com/apps/StoryMapCrowdsource/index.html?appid=19f5247b5bd043dda9a25b22c0919760.

Certeau, M. d. *The Pactice of Everyday Life* (Berkeley: University of California Press, 1984).

Condit, Celeste M. "Public Health Experts, Expertise, and Ebola: A Relational Theory of Ethos." *Rhetoric & Public Affairs* 22 (2), (2019): 177–215.

"Data Overview: Overview of the Drug Overdose Epidemic: Behind the Numbers." *Opioid Overdose, Centers for Disease Control and Prevention,* 2019, https://www.cdc.gov/drugoverdose/data/index.html.

Davisson, Amber. "Beyond the Borders of Red and Blue States: Google Maps as a Site of Rhetorical Invention in the 2008 Presidential Election." *Rhetoric and Public Affairs*, 14 (1), (2011): 119.

Dow, Bonnie J. "The Function of Epideictic and Deliberative Strategies in Presidential Crisis Rhetoric." *Western Journal of Speech Communication* 53 (Summer), (1989): 296.

"Ending America's Opioid Crisis." *Whitehouse.gov,* 2020, https://www.whitehouse.gov/opioids/.

Entman, R. M. "Framing: Toward Clarification of a Fractured Paradigm." *Journal of Communication* 43 (4), (1993): 51–58.

Ferrell, Ashley P. "'Righting Past Wrongs': Rhetorical Disidentification and Historical Reference in Response to Philadelphia's Opioid Epidemic." *Rhetoric & Public Affairs* 22 (4), (2019): 533–68.

Finkelman, Elizabeth M., and J. Michael McGinnis. "The Emergence of an Epidemic." In *A Public Health Guide to Ending the Opioid Epidemic*, edited by Jay C. Butler, and Michael R. Fraser (Oxford: Oxford University Press, 2019).

Flanigan, Andrew J. "The Impact of Contemporary Communication and Information Technologies on Police Organizations." In *Law Enforcement, Communication, and Community*, edited by Howard Giles (Philadelphia, PA: John Benjamins Publishing Company, 2002), 85–105.

Fleishman, Jeffrey. "Documentary Films Explore the Despair of America's Heroin and Opioid Epidemic." *The Los Angeles Times*, July 6, 2018, https://www.latimes.com/entertainment/movies/la-ca-opioids-documentaries-20180706-story.html.

Foster, Stephanie, Erica Adams, Ian Dunn, and Andrew Dent. "Geographic Information System Data: Epidemic Intelligence Service." *Centers for Disease Control,* December 13, 2018, https://www.cdc.gov/eis/field-epi-manual/chapters/GIS-data.html.

Gfroerer, Joseph. *War Stories from the Drug Survey: How Culture, Politics, and Statistics Shaped the National Survey on Drug Use and Health* (Cambridge: Cambridge University Press, 2019).

Gonzalez, Robbie. "This App Maps Opioid Overdoses in Real Time: Opioid Overdoses Proliferate, Like a Disease. A New App Lets Health and Law Enforcement Officials Anticipate their Spread." *WIRED,* September 22, 2017, https://www.wired.com/story/baltimore-built-an-app-to-map-opioid-overdoses-in-real-time/.

Gross, Terry. "'Drug Dealer, M.D.': Misunderstandings and Good Intentions Fueled Opioid Epidemic." *Fresh Air-NPR,* December 15, 2016, https://www.npr.org/sections/health-shots/2016/12/15/505710073/drug-dealer-md-contends-that-well-meaning-docs-drove-the-opioid-epidemic.

Hedges, Peter. "'Ben Is Back' Writer-Director Peter Hedges Uncovers the Heroic Core of Broken Women." *Los Angeles Times,* December 18, 2018, https://www.latimes.com/entertainment/envelope/la-en-mn-writing-ben-is-back-20181203-story.html.

Heroin(e), directed by Elaine McMillion Sheldon (Los Angeles, CA: Netflix, 2017), Streaming.

"Heroin(e)," *Netflix Media Center,* 2017, https://media.netflix.com/en/only-on-netflix/80192445.

"High Intensity Drug Trafficking Areas (HIDTAs)." *United* States Drug Enforcement Administration, Department of Justice, 2019, https://www.dea.gov/hidta.

"Home," *ODMAP.*org, 2019, http://odmap.org/#home.

Ivancic, Sonia R. "Body Sovereignty and Body Liability in the Wake of an 'Obesity Epidemic': A Poststructural Analysis of the Soda Ban." *Health Communication* 33 (10), (2018): 1243–56.

Jensen, Robin E. "Improving Upon Nature: The Rhetorical Ecology of Chemical Language, Reproductive Endocrinology, and the Medicalization of Infertility." *Quarterly Journal of Speech* 101 (2), (2015): 329–53.

Joseph, Alli. "Dr. Sanjay Gupta on How Income Inequality is Making Us Stressed Out." *Salon*, March 24, 2019, https://www.salon.com/2019/03/24/dr-sanjay-gupta-on-how-income-inequality-is-making-us-stressed-out/.

Joseph, Elizabeth. "Purdue Pharma Files for Bankruptcy as Part of a $10 billion Agreement to Settle Opioid Lawsuits." *CNN,* September 16, 2019, https://www.cnn.com/2019/09/16/us/purdue-pharma-bankruptcy-filing/index.html.

Kaur, Harmeet. "The Opioid Epidemic was Already a National Crisis. COVID-19 Could be Making Things Worse." *CNN,* May 7, 2020. https://www.cnn.com/2020/05/07/health/opioid-epidemic-covid19-pandemic-trnd/index.html.

Kreps, Daniel. "Chris Cornell's Widow Breaks Silence on Singer's Death, 'Addiction.'" *Rolling Stone,* June 28, 2017, https://www.rollingstone.com/music/music-news/chris-cornells-widow-breaks-silence-on-singers-death-addiction-201345/.

Kristof, Nicholas D. and Sheryl WuDunn. *Tightrope: Americans Reaching for Hope* (New York: Alfred A. Knopf, 2020).

Kristof, Nicholas and Sheryl WuDunn. "Who Killed the Knapp Family?" *The New York Times,* January 9, 2020, https://nyti.ms/37Qan0A.

Lakoff, G. and M. Johnson. *Philosophy in the Flesh* (New York: Basic Books, 1999).

Lembke, Anna M. D. *Drug Dealer, MD: How Doctors were Duped, Patients Got Hooked, and Why It's So Hard to Stop* (Baltimore: Johns Hopkins University Press, 2016).

Lupton, Deborah. "Foucault and the Medicalisation Critique." In *Foucault, Health and Medicine,* edited by Alan Petersen and Robin Bunton (London: Routledge, 1997), 94–110.

Mackey-Kallis, Susan and Dan Hahn. "Who's to Blame for America's Drug Problem?: The Search for Scapegoats in the 'War on Drugs.'" *Communication Quarterly* 42 (1), (1994): 6.

"March 19, 2018: Remarks on Combating the Opioid Crisis." UVA Miller Center, 2019, https://millercenter.org/the-presidency/presidential-speeches/march-19-2018-remarks-combating-opioid-crisis.

Meier, Barry. "Tightening the Lid on Pain Prescriptions." *The New York Times*, April 8, 2012, https://alliance-primo.hosted.exlibrisgroup.com/permalink/f/e3ml1m/TN_gale_ofa285683281.

Nichols, Bill. *Introduction to Documentary* (Bloomington: Indiana University Press, 2010).

Nichols, Bill. "History, Myth, and Narrative in Documentary." *Film Quarterly* 41 (1), (1987): 16.

"ODMAP Implementation Examples." *ODMAP.org.* 2019, http://odmap.org/#home.

Olson, Lester C., Cara A. Finnegan, and Diane S. Hope. "Introduction." In *Visual Rhetoric: A Reader in Communication and American Culture,* edited by Lester C. Olson, Cara A. Finnegan, and Diane S. Hope (Thousand Oaks, CA: Sage, 2008).

One Nation Under Stress: Deaths of Despair in the United States, directed by Marc Levin and Daphne Pinkerson (New York: HBO Documentary Films, 2019), Streaming.

"Opioid Overdose Crisis." *National Institute on Drug Abuse,* May 27, 2020, https://www.drugabuse.gov/drug-topics/opioids/opioid-overdose-crisis.

"Overdose Death Rates." *National Institute on Drug Abuse,* January 2019, https://www.drugabuse.gov/related-topics/trends-statistics/overdose-death-rates.

Parshley, Lois. "The Pandemic May Fuel the Next Wave of the Opioid Crisis." *National Geographic,* April 21, 2020, https://apple.news/AP1p3R64ES9So4tBOR-pdVA.

Phillips, Kendall R. *Dark Directions: Romero, Craven, Carpenter, and the Modern Horror Film* (Carbondale: Southern Illinois University Press, 2012).

Plantinga, Carl R. *Moving Viewers American Film and the Spectator's Experience* (Berkeley: University of California Press, 2009).

Prelli, Lawrence. *Rhetorics of Display* (Columbia: University of South Carolina Press, 2006).

Price, Thomas E. "Secretary Price Announces HHS Strategy for Fighting Opioid Crisis." *National Rx Drug Abuse and Heroin Summit,* April 19, 2017, https://www.hhs.gov/about/leadership/secretary/speeches/2017-speeches/secretary-price-announces-hhs-strategy-for-fighting-opioid-crisis/index.html.

Rosenblum, Andrew, Lisa A. March, Herman Joseph, and Russell K. Portenoy "Opioids and the Treatment of Chronic Pain: Controversies, Current Status, and Future Directions." *Expert Clinical Psychopharmacology* 16 (5), (2008): 405–16.

Rosteck, Thomas and Thomas S. Frentz. "The Conversion of Lila Lipscomb in Fahrenheit 9/11." In *Michael Moore and the Rhetoric of Documentary*, edited by Thomas W. Benson and Brian J. Snee (Carbondale: Southern Illinois University Press, 2015), 181.

Roth, Nancy L. "Dismantling the Mosaic of Misery: Louis Sullivan's Paradoxic Rhetorical Vision." *Howard Journal of Communications* 4 (3), (1993): 234–48.

Russell, David, Kelly M. Thames, and Naomi J. Spence. "'It's So Scary How Common This Is Now:' Frames in Media Coverage of the Opioid Epidemic by Ohio Newspapers and Themes in Facebook User Reactions." *Information, Communication & Society* 22 (5), (2019): 702–8.

Scott, A. O. "*Ben is Back* Review: A Mother and Son Face the Horrors of Addiction." *The New York Times,* December 5, 2018, https://www.nytimes.com/2018/12/05/movies/ben-is-back-review.html.

Scutchfield, F. D., and C. William Keck. "Deaths of Despair: Why? What to Do?" *American Journal of Public Health* 107 (10), (2017): 1564–65.

Sisco King, Claire. "Rogue Waves, Remakes, and Resurrections: Allegorical Displacement and Screen Memory in *Poseidon*." *Quarterly Journal of Speech* 94 (4), (2008): 431.

"Spike Alerts." *ODMAP.org,* 2019, http://odmap.org/#home.

Stache, Lara C. *Breaking Bad: A Cultural History* (Lanham: Rowman & Littlefield, 2017).

Sturken, Marita. *Tangled Memories: The Vietnam War, the AIDS Epidemic, and the Politics of Remembering* (Berkeley: University of California Press, 1997).

"The ODMAP Initiative." *Comprehensive Opioid Abuse Program,* 2019, https://odmap.coapresources.org.

"The Opioid Crisis." *Ending America's Opioid Crisis, Whitehouse.gov,* accessed January 2020, https://www.whitehouse.gov/opioids/.

Tobias, Scott. "*Ben is Back:* Well-Acted Addiction Drama Loses Its Way." *NPR,* December 6, 2018, https://www.npr.org/2018/12/06/673324119/ben-is-back-well-acted-addiction-drama-loses-its-way.

Vanguri, Star Medzerian. “Toward a Rhetorical Onomastics.” In *Rhetorics of Names and Naming,* edited by Star Medzerian Vanguri (New York: Routledge, 2016), 1.

Vivian, Bradford. “Witnessing Time: Rhetorical Form, Public Culture, and Popular Historical Education.” *Rhetoric Society Quarterly* 44 (3), (2014): 213.

Warnick, Barbara and David Heineman. *Rhetoric Online: The Politics of New Media* (New York: Peter Lang, 2012).

Welhausen, Candice A. “Power and Authority in Disease Maps: Visualizing Medical Cartography Through Yellow Fever Mapping.” *Journal of Business and Technical Communication* 29 (3), (2015): 261.

“West Virginia Opioid Summary.” *National Institute on Drug Abuse,* March 2019, https://www.drugabuse.gov/opioid-summaries-by-state/west-virginia-opioid-summary.

Wilkins, Karin. “Mapping Fear and Danger in Global Space.” *International Communication Gazette* 71(7), (2009): 561.

Willis, Erin, and Chad Painter. “The Needle and the Damage Done: Framing the Heroin Epidemic in the Cincinnati Enquirer.” *Health Communication* 34 (6), (2019): 661–71.

Wyatt, Ronald M.D., M.H.A. “Pain and Ethnicity.” *American Medical Association Journal of Ethics,* May 2013. https://journalofethics.ama-assn.org/article/pain-and-ethnicity/2013-05.

Yartey, Franklin Nii Amankwah. “The Critical Condition of Rhetorical Choices.” *Journal of International Communication* 21 (2), (2015): 226–40.

Zelizer, Barbie. “Finding Aids to the Past: Bearing Personal Witness to Traumatic Public Events.” *Media, Culture & Society* 24 (5), (2002): 698.

Zoorob, Michael J. and Jason L. Salemi. “Bowling Alone, Dying Together: The Role of Social Capital in Mitigating the Drug Overdose Epidemic in the United States.” *Drug and Alcohol Dependence* 173 (2017): 1–9.

Index

addict, 35, 47, 48, 59, 112
addiction, 4, 5, 9, 18, 19, 20, 26, 30, 34, 35, 38, 47, 49, 50, 51, 53, 56, 57, 58, 65, 73, 74, 78, 82, 93, 102, 110, 111, 113, 114, 115, 122, 123, 126, 128

Ben is Back, 13, 47–62, 122, 125
biomedical model, 97, 98, 100, 101, 102

China, 68, 69, 76, 80
chronic pain, 19, 92, 123, 126, 127
chronic pain management debate, 2, 14, 107–20, 127
criminality frame, 9, 121, 122
consubstantiality, 50

Democrats, 73, 74, 80, 81
deaths of despair, 2, 12, 13, 17, 18, 20, 22, 30, 31, 40, 43, 44, 56, 67, 91, 92, 126
doctor, 19, 27, 28, 39, 40, 41, 42, 52, 53, 56, 70, 112, 115, 116, 125, 126
documentary films, 13, 25–46, 124

epideictic rhetoric, 64, 65, 69, 90
epidemic:
crack-cocaine epidemic, 3, 8, 13, 22, 57, 67, 121
HIV/AIDS epidemic, 3, 8, 9, 10, 22, 23
obesity epidemic, 9, 11

fentanyl, 8, 26, 33, 35, 43, 69, 75, 78, 98, 99, 108, 126

governmental responses, 1, 2, 3, 6, 8, 9, 12, 13, 63–86, 87–106
Gupta, Sanjay M. D., 1, 27, 30, 38–44

Hedges, Lucas, 47, 48, 125
Hedges, Peter, 13, 47, 48, 50, 57, 60, 61
heroin, 1, 5, 8, 20, 21, 25, 33, 35, 59, 61, 73, 74, 87, 98, 99, 109, 121, 126
Heroin(e), 2, 25–46, 49, 125
HIDTA (High-Intensity Drug Trafficking agency), 2, 81, 87–106, 124
hydrocodone, 39, 42

identification, 28, 29, 36, 40, 48, 50, 51, 52, 53, 54, 56

legal framing, 66, 68, 69, 70, 75, 76, 78, 79, 80

MAT (medication-assisted treatment), 20, 82

maps, 87–106, 124
media framing, 14, 111, 112
medicalization, 3, 4, 5, 6, 9, 14, 27, 36, 40, 41, 55, 56, 58, 70, 75, 79, 81, 82, 89, 93, 95, 97, 98, 99, 100, 102, 111, 112, 114, 116, 117, 118, 121, 122, 123, 124, 125, 126
Mexico, 68, 69, 70, 80
mother, 39, 47, 48, 49, 50, 51, 52, 53, 54, 55, 57, 58, 61, 125

Naloxone, 2, 5, 32, 34, 35, 42, 55, 56, 59, 60, 88, 92, 93, 94, 95, 97, 100, 101, 102, 103, 124, 126
narrative, 9, 21, 23, 27, 30, 48, 49, 50, 51, 55, 56, 61, 78, 93, 101, 112, 113, 114, 116, 117, 123, 125
  narrative arc, 27, 32, 42, 43, 112
  narrative conversions, 31, 38

ODMAP (Overdose Detection Mapping Application Program), 14, 81, 87–106, 124
One Nation Under Stress: Deaths of Despair in the United States, 2, 13, 25–46
opioid epidemic:
  background, 17–24, 25–27, 63, 91–92, 107–10, 121–22, 126–28
OxyContin, 19, 42, 109, 113, 127

pain, 1, 17, 19, 20, 21, 22, 42, 44, 51, 92, 98, 107, 108–120
painkiller, 78, 109, 112, 117, 118
pharmaceutical companies, 11, 19, 55, 79, 109, 110, 111, 113, 114, 115, 116, 117, 118, 122, 124, 125, 126, 127
popular culture, 1, 12, 40, 67, 122, 127
popular media, 6, 13, 14, 48, 108, 122, 124
prescriber, 19, 39, 108, 109, 111, 112
presidential rhetoric, 63–86
public health frame, 3, 4, 6, 11, 14, 22, 27, 40, 41, 55, 65, 74, 81, 82, 89, 92, 97, 99, 101, 121, 123, 124, 125
public health crisis/emergency, 1, 2, 4, 7, 10, 18, 27, 63, 64, 65, 70, 80, 95, 100, 107, 111, 116, 118, 122, 123, 127
Purdue Pharma, 1, 109, 110, 113, 114, 127

Rader, Jan, 27, 30, 31–38, 41, 42
representative anecdote, 12, 14, 76, 116
Republican, 73, 80
Roberts, Julia, 47, 48, 49, 53, 125

sound, 52
stigma, 5, 6, 20, 25, 26, 48, 78, 82, 122, 123, 124
synecdoche, 2, 27, 29, 32, 33, 34, 36, 37, 40, 44, 47, 48, 49, 53, 54, 57, 58, 59, 60, 68, 71, 72, 78, 89, 97, 103, 111, 112, 113, 115, 118, 124, 125
synecdochal, 27, 36, 44, 50, 69, 113, 125

testimony, 27, 28, 29, 34, 35, 41, 97, 115, 116
Trump, Donald, 2, 18, 63–86, 122

victimage, 66, 80
visual rhetoric, 25–62, 87–106
visualization, 88, 89

war on drugs, 5, 7, 9, 13, 14, 22, 65, 66, 71, 81, 82, 92, 121, 122, 123

About the Author

Tiara K. Good is a faculty member in the Communication Studies Department at Western Oregon University.

www.ingramcontent.com/pod-product-compliance
Lightning Source LLC
LaVergne TN
LVHW091532200926
848483LV00002B/373